UNEXPECTED WELLNESS

A RADICALLY SIMPLE APPROACH TO
HEALTHY LIVING

Disclaimer:

The information contained within this text is not designed to diagnose, treat, or offer cures for conditions, diseases, or syndromes of any kind. While great care has been taken to ensure accuracy of the information presented, the authors cannot assume responsibility for the validity of all materials or the consequences of their use. Before making any changes or starting any health program it is always recommended to seek the counsel and approval from your regular physician.

"Thanks to the tips and daily practices in your book, I've been able to increase my energy level and feel more clear in my approach to wellness." - Jay Wright

"As a working mom, I don't have time to follow every new fitness and diet trend. Dr. Kevin and Dr. April recommend clear, simple, affordable lifestyle changes that anyone can make. *Unexpected Wellness* is essential reading for everyone who wants to cut through the hype and truly take charge of their health."
– Maria Veres, Best Selling Author

"I loved Dr. Kevin and Dr. April Morford's book. It was very simple and fun reading. Kept me engaged and eager for the next step. I loved all the simple ways they have for me to implement a healthier lifestyle." - Patricia Howard

"Drs. Kevin and April Morford have helped me get back the appreciation for the role that health, and especially my energy level, plays in my life and business. Just one of these tips can change your life." -Tim Wolf

"The information in this book is easy to use. It provides an insightful contribution to the understanding of how to achieve wellness through mind, body and spirit." - J. Reed, E.I., C.H.T.P.

Acknowledgments

Thank you to the incredible people who have shared their stories and their knowledge with us whether it be through academics, clinical practice, or personal experience. Special gratitude to our parents, whose patience and understanding along with unshakeable faith made any of this possible. Jay Wright willfully and expertly helped turn this into an actual book with edits and insights. Maria Veres went above and beyond by providing the knowledge and patience to answer our questions and help us move this book to publishing. Suellen Miller provided a platform for the development of these ideas by accepting articles for her monthly newsletter. Tim Wolf gave us input on making this book marketable and impactful. Jerome Braggs was instrumental in moving us forward and providing inspiration. Lastly, our deep gratitude to our teacher, coach, guide and friend Dr. Sue Morter and her "village people" for openly welcoming us into their world where we have experienced true depth in our own personal growth.

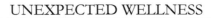

To our parents, who have lovingly supported us through it all.

And to our daughter, Alyssa.

Table of Contents

Introduction

Albert Einstein said, *"If you can't explain it simply, you don't understand it well enough."* Looking at our healthcare system today and the way we generally approach our health, it seems very few people truly understand what it takes to be healthy, vital, free, and joyful about their body and their life.

This book is created to reverse that. It is designed to allow continual progress through taking easy, small steps that lead to greater health and vibrancy. Following the twenty-one recommendations within this text will provide you an amazing, solid platform from which you can build towards a body that supports your ambitions, drives you towards your goals, and provides the energy needed to strive for and reach the life of your dreams.

We do this by providing simple concepts that can be implemented immediately and begin to impact your body today! All without having to turn your life upside down spending hours at the gym or having to follow confusing diet plans that are tasteless and boring.

Honestly, the fact that these ideas are so basic and yet so effective almost always exceeds people's expectations. In the end they find themselves feeling an unexpected level of health and vitality using a radically simple approach and wonder why no else ever told them it could be this way. These easy to apply, daily action steps surprisingly led them to new levels of *Unexpected Wellness!*

How do we know it works? Every one of these steps is part of our personal lives on a very regular basis. While some of them come in handy in particular situations, others have their place as a daily habit. We practice them knowing through our own experiences how powerful they are. We've seen the changes in ourselves and recognized how our energy and health improves following these rules. Staying on course and continually using these simple steps to transforming health has provided us with greater mental clarity, an abundance of energy, and deeper levels of joy. It has been a key part of our ability to teach clients, treat patients, and speak at conferences while having the vitality and freedom to be with one another and spend valuable time with our daughter. It has literally kept us out of doctor's offices for over a decade.

The changes you hope to see for yourself are available to you through these pages. Whatever your current state of health, no matter your weight or history, the opportunity to create a body that supports your ideal life is right here. We won't guarantee six pack abs or losing 30 pounds in 30 days. But we will guarantee that in one month with continual use of these basic concepts you will notice more energy, joy, and freedom in your life.

Actually, those typical promises are a major reason we created this book in the first place. We grew tired of all the gimmicks and games being played. Special drinks, seven day plans, skinny body wraps, etc. are found around every corner. The number of people we know personally who have tried a variety of these programs and products is quite large. Those that do so aren't dumb. They aren't poor gullible souls being duped. They are making honest attempts at improving their lives searching for answers and willing to try anything to make it work for them.

Unfortunately, most of what you find on bookshelves and down grocery aisles isn't designed for sustained success. It's built for rapid results dependent on outside factors and almost always reliant on their particular product. If you get any results at all, they're usually here today and gone tomorrow. This is how we've created a cycle of yo-yo dieting and extreme workouts that lead to pain and frustration.

If you want positive, long lasting changes in your health it's time to get back to doing what's real and effective. Something that empowers you to make positive changes that become healthy habits and lead to actual transformations. No nonsense about using this special drink or taking that special pill. Just the real factors needed for real results that we've honed in on through a combined 30 years of clinical practice, personal study and continued refinement.

Will you lose weight? Almost assuredly. Will you get tone and firm muscles? Certainly. Will you get mental clarity and peace of mind? We sure do. Will you build a stronger immune system able to fight off diseases helping you fend of sickness and recover from illness more quickly? Absolutely. Will you get more energy to play, laugh, work, dance, and enjoy life? Yes.

But you must act. Which is why we strive to keep it so simple. *Simplicity leads to Action!*

*****

"Where there is confusion, momentum halts." – Jay Wright

There are a couple pieces of advice we'd like to share with you before you start reading and putting into practice these simple steps.

First, while the steps in here are very simple in nature, the application of some of them may be challenging. We've provided ideas from a range of important areas that directly impact your health. From diet to exercise to thoughts, these steps in and of themselves are not hard to do. But they can often be difficult to use because it takes some level of introspection and time to learn and fully understand what these ideas mean or why they make a difference in your body's highest functioning.

You'll find some changes come easily while others may come with discomfort and struggle. And while it is often very easy to start with a high level of motivation, it's only in turning these practices into daily habits that you'll achieve long term success. Don't quit or become discouraged. A single action has more power than a million doubts. Just start and changes will happen.

Secondly, one of the interesting catches to these steps is that some are almost so ridiculously simple they are easy to disregard. This takes us back to Einstein's quote about simplicity. In an age where we have trained ourselves to recognize the use of high tech gadgets, lab generated foods, and fad diets as the means to attaining health, we've started overlooking the simplicity that is required for us to take care of our bodies and experience true health and wellness.

Don't fall into this trap! Each of the steps we provide is done so with great care because it is through our personal experience and working with thousands of clients that we have found the foundational keys to extraordinary health. Their simplicity is the greatest benefit of all. If you doubt that something as simple as breathing properly can alter your entire body, try it for a week before casting it aside. Conduct your own experiments with each step to understand their value.

As a first step in this process, we highly recommend that you begin by identifying your intentions for your health. Write them down and place them somewhere you will see them every day. Search into the deeper meaning of your intentions to find inspiration.

For example, weight loss is the most common intention people choose. But what is the value behind the weight loss? Do you want to have more energy? Feel more confident? Be able to play with your kids or grandkids? Identifying the true reasons that weight loss is important to you provides an ideal to push you onward even when the scale isn't showing you progress. Searching for those deeper reasons lets you know the "why" of weight loss and when times get tough, act as the inspiration to keep going. Set the intentions based on the deeper inspirations rather than the superficial goal. No matter what your intention is, keeping a heart-felt reason for it is incredibly powerful.

Speaking of intentions, it is *our intention* that this book be read section by section not cover to cover. Read through one of the recommendations and work on applying it into your life before moving on to the next one. Give each topic at least a day, maybe a week, to notice its effects. Whether you do one each day for 21 days, or do the same one for 21 days, you will feel a difference. However you apply them, continue to add each step in line. Find a system that works for you and as you notice changes in your body and mind take another step in fueling that positive growth. Watch 21 days become 210 days, and you'll be amazed at how far you've come. Watch a conscious decision to implement a plan for just 21 days become a true healthy habit.

At the end of each section we've provided action steps that help you identify precisely how you can utilize the recommendation you've just finished reading. It may be beneficial to write them down and carry them with you on a sticky note or as a note in your phone. That way you'll continually be reminded of the changes you're working on making. Putting these action steps into practice is the only way you will create positive changes. Learning how to make them part of your everyday life will allow you to make permanent changes that provide continued freedom.

Lastly, know that with this information we've still only scratched the surface of the true depth available for extraordinary health. But instead of overwhelming ourselves with drastic and difficult changes, we found that for ourselves and for our clients, breaking these big ideas into simple action steps was the key to good, sustainable results.

We are **not** intent on you *knowing* these steps, but on your ability to *implement* them. The information you will be reading can guide you through transforming your health in every area of your life.

True health, a life filled with inspiration, is only achieved through the full integration of every part of you…..mind, body, and soul. Every recommendation we have made is designed to help you achieve exactly that. As you read on and apply these action steps, give thanks for the time and opportunity to honor these three parts of yourself. And know that in doing so, you've already taken the most important step of all…..getting started.

Chapter 1

Get More of that Magic Elixir of Life....Water

When it comes to simple ways of improving your health, this one is probably pretty obvious. We've all been told on a regular basis since we were children that we should drink eight glasses of water every day. The problem is that we still don't follow that advice and likewise don't drink enough of the purifying elixir. Part of the reason is that our choices regarding drinks has such variety now that water just gets overlooked or considered boring.

It's important to make sure you are nourishing your body with plenty of water every single day. Here are three ways that we have found are extremely helpful in increasing our water intake and getting more of this magic elixir of life into our day.

First, each morning after you've risen and used the restroom go to the kitchen and drink a tall glass of nice, cool water. This simple habit awakens and feeds every cell of the body. It activates the digestive organs, gets the blood pumping, and refreshes muscles. You begin the day by flushing out waste, restoring energy within your cells, and waking up the brain. As simple as this is, we've found it incredibly helpful not only for making sure we drink enough during the day, but in getting the morning and the day off to a powerful start. Quite often we can feel it wash away early morning grogginess and get our minds set for what lies ahead. Your body will thank for building the habit-muscle of starting each day with a glass of water.

> *A tall glass of water first thing in the morning has been one of the best habits we've formed.*

Second, take water with you. This is easier today than it's ever been. You can buy water in any store or you can get your own personal water bottle and fill it regularly to take with you wherever you go. We have stainless steel water bottles with tight lids that we fill up and take nearly everywhere. Only when we're going to a restaurant and know we'll be having water there do we ever not have water with us. The simple fact is that having water available leads to us drink considerably more. It's easy to almost unconsciously reach for a water bottle sitting at your desk and sip on it throughout the day. But if there's not one nearby, it never fails that we'll go hours without it. Out of sight, out of mind. Simple? Yes. Effective? YES!

The third tip really comes down to making water something you'll look forward to drinking. It has become incredibly easy to get any variety of different drinks at gas stations and drive thru windows. And, honestly, a glass of sweet tea, soda, or coffee often sound far more appetizing than a few glugs of water. This is is why we add something to our water in times when we start getting bored. Squeezing some fresh lemon or lime, dropping in a couple cucumber slices (which sounds weird but is surprisingly refreshing), and even putting a slice of orange in provides a nice, subtle touch of flavor that makes drinking water far less dull. It helps with stopping that feeling that you're missing out on something sweet and tasty by drinking plain old water. Now you get to experience a shot of flavor, a few added nutrients, and the benefits of water, all at once.

Why is this really all that crucial? The facts that the human body is around 70% water is traditionally the logic people tend to use as the major reason for regular water intake. Even if it's true, which it is, that line of reasoning doesn't get people to start drink what they should. Just saying it'll make you healthier doesn't seem to help either. But consider some of the benefits below and see if there's one or more you'd like to have more of in your life.

Here are just a few changes people notice when they start drinking more water: *clear skin, relaxed muscles, reduced pain and smooth moving joints, better digestion, mental clarity, improved circulation, abundant energy, and (one almost everyone wants help with) weight loss[1]*.

Any of that sound nice? All of that seem ideal? You get all of that with this first tip. But there's still more.

The quick act of taking even a sip of water effects every part of the body. A friend of mine, Dr. Jason Redler, studied biochemistry as an undergrad. He relayed to me an experiment they did tracking where in the body water goes whenever we take a drink. The results were amazing. What they found was that whenever we take water into the body, every single cell takes a collective sip. Each cell gets a fresh rush of refreshing H_2O that boosts its own, individual cellular functions.

One major benefit of this is increased energy. If you have a tendency to feel sluggish and tired in the middle or end of your day pay close attention. Water is a critical nutrient used in the process of making energy in your body. Each cell requires it to go through the chemical reactions that build energy in a clean and efficient manner. Which means that when you're feeling run down, instead of reaching for another energy drink, you should be reaching for water.

You already know this is important. Maybe you've learned a couple more reasons why. And if you've been struggling with weight loss or chronic fatigue, this may be the foundational principle that you need to implement to begin your transformation. Stay on course and begin to notice the benefit of better hydration by following these three simple recommendations and applying them into your day.

Get more of that elixir of life... water

Simple Health Action Steps

1. Drink a glass of cool, refreshing water first thing in the morning.

2. Take a reusable bottle of water with you wherever you go.

3. Add lemon, cucumber, orange, or some other fruit to add flavor and overcome boredom. This has an added benefit of offering some detoxification value at the same time.

Chapter 2

Boost Energy and Bust Stress: Practice Deep Breathing

On a beautiful summer day I was a typical kid outside playing football with my friends. The yard next to our house was large enough to let us run around, but it was still surrounded by trees. During one play the ball was thrown just beyond my route. Adjusting to make the play I headed directly towards a tree branch sitting almost perfectly at chest level. The moment I hit that branch I felt the air forced from my lungs. The panic and awkward gasping took forever to subside as I fought the feeling of suffocation. Regaining my breath was the biggest relief I'd ever experienced.

Usually the first impression regarding directions for better breathing, without thinking about it, is dismissive. Why do we need to practice deep breathing, or practice breathing at all? We do it on our own every moment of every day without even thinking about it, right?

There are two major reasons that a practice of deep breathing is an important part of vibrant health.…..*stress* and *energy*.

Let's look at stress first. Stress is a major irritant in the body. It stimulates a part of the nervous system called our "Fight or Flight" system. This is the protective aspect of us that senses danger and then prepares us to either fight or run, habitually weighing and considering the options on what it thinks provides our best chance for survival. While this is helpful in life threatening situations like being attacked by a bear, it becomes harmful continually running in the absence of an imminent threat. But that's exactly what happens to almost everyone on a daily basis. It often acts as a subconscious loop playing in the background that we don't even know is rolling.

Our major threats to survival that our furthest ancestors had to deal with are rarely an issue any more. But we've replaced them with the stresses of everyday life. The bears and tigers of our ancestor's days have become the to-do lists of today. Between taking care of the kids, going to work, meeting deadlines, paying bills, getting groceries and making dinner, finding time to get to the gym, and spending quality time with the family; many are stretched to the max. This puts us under constant mental and physiological stress. We worry endlessly. And the results are easy to see.

When the body gets stressed, it changes its physiology. Your heart rate and blood pressure increase, and your breathing becomes more rapid. Muscles tense while digestion slows. Blood flow is shifted from life-sustaining functions to survival ones. (After all, you don't need to worry about digesting dinner if you *are* dinner.) We even shift activity in the brain from a rational, logical process to a scanning, vigilant mindset on the lookout for more danger. In fact, the list of changes in the body directly correlates to what we see as the most prevalent health conditions people suffer from today!

Do you suffer from high blood pressure, breathing problems like asthma, poor digestion, sore muscles, achy joints, mental fatigue, inability to focus, frequent illness, weight gain, lack of energy, or headaches? Each of these are directly linked to the stress reaction in the body. Over time these changes in the basic way your body works causes the various cells to break down and become diseased. Or as we say "dis-ease"…a lack of ease.

Related to stress but deserving of its own time is the aspect of energy. Your body can create energy in two ways; with oxygen and without it. One is incredibly efficient and creates a high amount of energy with little waste product left over. The other is helpful in providing quick fuel but only provides a small amount of energy and leaves behind a nasty byproduct. Can you guess which is which?

If you guessed that the method utilizing high levels of oxygen is the more efficient one, you're right. We get around *six times* as much energy when the cellular engines, called mitochondria, have oxygen available to produce that energy! Strip or drastically reduce the oxygen available and the energy production goes down while the waste levels go up. You feel that waste product as sore muscles, achy joints, and drained energy even after a good night of sleep.

As strange as this sounds, we've spoken at conferences and coached individuals about this simple technique. It's really that powerful and obviously ridiculously simple. One client, Karen, uses these simple techniques to alleviate pain in her low back, calm herself down during exams in her nursing program, and find the energy to go to school, work, and care for two kids....as a single mom! She was just as surprised as anyone how much this worked.

So how do you combat the ill effects of stress AND get to boost your energy at the same time? Deep breathing. Specifically, deep breathing with your belly. Test yourself and then practice this regularly to make sure you're getting the most of out of every breath.

Place your hand on your belly button and breathe out as much as you can. When you begin to inhale, notice if your belly button is pushing out while you breathe in. Then as you exhale see if that belly button squeezes back in as you breathe out. This is the natural motion of the belly with each breath in relation to the anatomy and physiology of the body. If you're not breathing like this, you're missing out and denying your cells oxygen to combat stress and boost energy.

Again: Breathe in – Belly goes out. Breathe out – Belly goes in.

Check yourself with this practice regularly. Especially do it when you're upset! Times of high stress are when we commonly alter our breathing pattern and actually feed into the stress making it worse. If you only catch yourself once a day, what a great start! Soon it'll become once an hour then maybe even every few minutes. Cut the anxiety and create more clean energy by taking a few deep breaths. It really is that simple and that powerful.

Practice of deep breathing

Simple Health Action Steps:

1. Test your breathing right now to see if you are following the correct belly in/belly out pattern.

2. Notice during stressful times at work, in the car, or at home to see if your breathing pattern changes under those conditions.

3. Set up times in your day, maybe even put reminders in your cell phone, to stop and take a couple deep breaths to restore your energy and diminish stress.

Chapter 3

Poisons in Your Pantry: Decoding Nutrition on Food Packaging

During our schooling we both took a number of nutrition courses. That of course led to us being far pickier at the grocery store. We made one trip to Walmart looking for bread that was free of harmful ingredients. After an hour in just the bread aisle, we walked out empty handed. That began an intensive project in deciphering how to really find healthy food while shopping for groceries. And where it led us was quite a surprise.

On all boxed, canned, and packaged foods, there is white box that contains the nutrition information listing the important details of the nutritional products that are contained in that food. This is where you find information including calories, sodium, carbohydrates, fats, and proteins. Near it is also where you find the ingredients needed to make that product.

The nutrition information in the white box was put on packaging to make reading and understanding the label very simple and easy. In doing so, it was believed that choosing healthier options would be easier for the average consumer (i.e. you and I). They even did things like adding percentages associated with what percent of your diet that particular item will provide. For example, you might find that a bag of potato chips has 25% of your total sodium intake for the day. Though this information is very helpful and can act at least as a deterrent for buying low quality food, it seems like the most important information is ignored.

This key information is the ingredient list.

Here is how our family chooses foods while we're at the grocery store. We spend little time reading the white and black "Nutrition Facts" box. Honestly, we couldn't tell you the calories or grams of fat that is found in a large portion of our groceries. Our focus when deciding on food is the ingredients. If the ingredients contained in the food are healthy ingredients and free from harmful products then we choose that food. If we're comparing two different types of cookies, we don't look at how many calories, grams of sodium, or amount of fat is in them. We compare their ingredient lists and choose the one made with products that are more naturally healthy, and support our bodies.

How can we view it this way? Because the concern is not over *calories* but over *nutrients*. If we consume enough nutrients our bodies get all they need to feel good and function great. After a quality meal, our bodies signal to us that we have eaten enough food (calories) because it's gotten the raw materials to function optimally (nutrients). There's no need to go and seek out more calories in an attempt to satisfy our nutrient needs. On the other hand, if we are starving our body of nutrients while continuing to feed it endless calories, the body *still keeps asking for more food* (adding more calories) in an attempt to get the nutrients it is craving. Quality nutrients are reflected in the ingredients. Food labels focus on the quantity of the product. We choose quality over quantity. We also haven't been to a doctor in over ten years. Coincidence? I think not.

> **Ingredient lists are better reflections of food quality and health than the "Nutrition Facts."**

The list of ingredients is typically found underneath the nutrition label on almost all food packages (but not always so there are occasions that you'll have to look around to find them). Here are a few general rules for looking at the ingredient list and determining which foods will be Health Boosting vs. Health Busting.

- If you can't pronounce it, put it back on the shelf – this reflects the likelihood that the food product is more chemical than actual food. It's generally best to avoid it. (Ex. Sodium Stearoyl Lactylate)

- Search for these three words and AVOID them! *Modified, Artificial, and Hydrogenated. Modified* reflects genetically modified foods which the health community is hotly debating over whether or not they're safe for us to eat, even in small amounts[1]. But it's kind of interesting that many other countries are banning GMO foods[2].

Artificial can highlight artificial sweeteners. These are getting sneaky and they are coming out with new names to hide these toxic substances in your labels. If you see artificial anything we highly recommend skipping it. Also look for these terms that are other names for artificial sweeteners: Acesulfame K, Sucralose, MSG, Aspartame, and Amino Sweet. (See later chapter for more info and resources.)

Hydrogenated highlights the presence of trans-fats. Even if you read the fancy black and white box proudly proclaiming "No Trans Fats," if you see hydrogenated (especially with the world *partially* in front of it), that food likely has trans fats in it. Explaining why the FDA lets that happen is another discussion.

- Foods with the fewest ingredients will also usually be some of the best. It tells you the food has not been overly treated or altered and is close to its pure form. We try to find foods with seven (7) items or less on the ingredient list.

- Look for real, whole food. Apple sauce should be made with real apples. Potato chips made with potatoes. Spaghetti sauce ought to have tomatoes mostly. These should be seen first on the ingredients list. For example, if you're shopping for ketchup, be sure that tomatoes are the first (and therefore most abundant) ingredient and not something like sugar or high fructose corn syrup. Seems common sense, but when you start reading labels it'll shock you what's out there.

Poisons in your pantry

Simple Health Action Steps:

1.   Read the ingredient list when grocery shopping, not just the nutrition label. Don't trust the claims on the front of the product.

2.   Avoid products riddled with fake chemicals that typically have long names. Discard modified, artificial, and hydrogenated.

3.   Find food that is made with natural, real products. Make sure it's the first item listed in the ingredients list meaning it is the most abundant ingredient. (i.e. Whole wheat bread should have "whole wheat" as the first ingredient listed)

Chapter 4

The Many Uses of Coconut Oil

Do you remember the beloved movie The Wizard of Oz? Dorothy runs into a character called the Tin Man who cries for assistance with his oil can. After a few squirts he comes to life loosening his joints and happily dancing down the yellow brick road. Turns out the Tin Man had it right for us too. Oil serves our bodies as well. And one of the best is coconut oil.

Coconut oil gets a bad rap because of one major thing; it is a saturated fat. But this is not as bad as we are taught to think. Coconut oil has a different profile and molecular structure than other saturated fats which allows the body to use it more readily. Scientifically it is classified as a Medium Chain Fatty Acid (MCFA). As a smaller fatty acid, coconut oil is easier for our bodies to use for energy. We don't pack away coconut oil like we do other heavy fats that come from sources like pork and margarine. So the concern over clogging arteries is very low. Here are some other things about coconut oil you should know.

A report in the Journal of Nutrition in 2002 found that people using coconut oil stored less fat in their abdomen compared to those who did not use coconut oil[1]. And in 2009 the journal *Lipids* found similar results where people who used coconut oil burned a higher ratio of fat during weight loss[2]. Some reports say that it may even speed up metabolism! You could burn higher levels of fat, in areas where it tends to hang out and drive people crazy, while stimulating your metabolism. Seems like a pretty good deal to me! But we're not done.

Dr. Weston A. Price, known for studying how nutrition played a role in health outside of the lab, saw groups of indigenous people in the South Pacific eating high levels of coconut. They looked healthy with trim bodies despite eating a diet so high in fat our Western world would blush just thinking about it[3]. A study done way back in 1981 published in the American Journal of Clinical Nutrition also found that these people had very healthy cardiovascular health even with diets high in saturated fat[4]. Findings exactly opposite of almost everything we're told about eating fat today.

And yet the story is not yet complete. Coconut oil is also rich in many other health producing compounds. One of these compounds is the immune builder Lauric Acid, which helps fend off viruses, bacteria and other infectious critters. Numerous studies have shown that coconut oil is useful in lessening pain, decreasing inflammation and even reducing itching[5, 6].

How do we use it in our home? It's only one of about three or four oils that we cook with, ever. And among those we have it is the most commonly used hands down. It can replace butter as a spread on toast, serve as oil for baking, is great for greasing cookware, and does all of this with very mild taste so your food doesn't come out tasting like coconut all the time.

Outside of the kitchen it serves as a lotion that nourishes and soothes the skin. We've even found a recipe for deodorant that can be made with coconut oil and other products that works really well, even in intense heat, but doesn't contain harsh chemicals like many name brand deodorants. It's used as make-up remover, helps speed recovery from sunburn, and may even be useful as part of toothpaste.

Do note that this oil seems strange because it can quickly change from a liquid to solid and vice versa. Its chemical profile allows it to move between the solid and liquid form very easily right around room temperature. So in the winter it'll appear solid and over the warm summer tend to be more liquid. In either state, it's available for all the same uses.

Needless to say, the stuff is incredible. It is a primary staple in our house that has found its way into many parts of our lives. Now it's hard to imagine our home without it.

Many uses of coconut oil

Simple Health Action Step:

1.   Find organic, cold-pressed, extra virgin coconut oil and start using it in a variety of dishes. Remember that it may be either liquid or solid, but if it meets the criteria just mentioned you're good to go!

2.   Use coconut oil as skin lotion, give yourself a mini-massage with it, and add a drop of essential oil to enhance its effect.

3.   Try coconut oil as the spread on your toast replacing margarine or butter. Substitute it for shortening or other oil in your muffins and cookies. It can be used in a 1:1 ratio just like the other common cooking oils.

Chapter 5

Getting Back to Basics

One of the issues many people experience when trying to improve their health is confusion over what is true and useful versus what's just a giant waste of time. Different outlets provide differing opinions and information. Today you watch a report on NBC that promotes running as the greatest form of exercise. Tomorrow CBS tells you running leads to more deaths each year than car accidents. Okay, I'm exaggerating, but this kind of thing happens all the time. How do you know what's true and who do you trust? Even doctors disagree on what's healthy and what's not!

Unfortunately, clients have told us their confusion often leads to them simply giving up. It became too frustrating to sort out what works and what doesn't. It was easier to throw their hands in the air and say forget it. Heck, even as practicing doctors we find it confusing to sort through all the data to figure out what's true and what's false. This led to the important realization that the best advice is to K.I.S.S

– Keep It Simple Silly. When we applied it for ourselves, the results were profound.

The basics of a healthy lifestyle boil down to the same things we were told to do back in grade school. Keeping it simple means eating fruits and veggies, having plenty of time to relax, getting the body moving with exercise or walks outside, and having quality family time. Trips to the grocery store can be simplified by spending most of your time shopping in the produce department. Instead of buying diet sodas, protein bars, tasteless "sugar-free" cookies, and gimmick food, keep it simple and buy an apple. Even if you don't have hours available to try out the newest exercise craze you can still keep your joints happy and muscles loose. Just go outside and walk the dog or play with your children. Ultimately, it is that simple!

One of the basics that our family has been implementing more of is eating together at the dinner table. We've even started decorating the table to make it nice to eat at and utilize it for more than a spot to hold mail, files from work, and random items thrown there when we walk in the door. This has had a number of positive effects.

Eating together leads to us sharing and talking for a long time reconnecting us with one another each day. We are more mindful of the food we eat, paying attention to actually enjoying our meal instead of mindlessly shoveling it in our mouths by the forkful hardly noticing the tastes, aromas, and visual appeal. It seems to even slow things down, taking the hectic lifestyle we often all live, and bringing peace and calm to the moment.

Another important simple act is daily reading. Spend time during the day, even a few minutes in the morning especially, to read something that engages your mind, providing inspiration and stimulating imagination. The calmness that comes with even ten minutes of quietly reading with a cup of coffee in hand is something you begin to cherish. It provides a sound platform for approaching your day and takes your mind off of the to-do list we have a tendency to start running through in our minds.

The basics of today are the same as they were 50 years ago. Sure, things have gotten more complicated, but keeping it simple is the key to success.

We know that life may seem too busy to do these things all the time. Certainly not every day. And believe me, we don't get to do these every single day. Life just doesn't always allow it. But it is important that you find ways to honor yourself and your basic needs daily. If dinner can't be had together at the table, you still apply simple appreciation for whatever and wherever you're eating with whomever you get to share it with, gratefully.

One habit we personally find ourselves locked into that doesn't benefit our health, relationships, or minds is television. We get caught using a movie as our "video babysitter" where we distract our daughter in an attempt to achieve our daily tasks. But does it have to be on all the time? Do our days need to revolve around favorite shows or sporting events? Again, we're just as guilty of this as anyone.

However, we recognize the impact just watching less TV can have. We've gotten rid of cable and found our time reading has grown exponentially. We play more, laugh more, share more, and get outside more. Mind-numbing TV time turns into a chance for growth, love, play, and fun. It's amazing how much free time you find yourself having when the TV doesn't control your day.

We estimate you can alter your current state of health by around 90% if you just make simple changes. The basics have been around for thousands of years and will remain true for thousands more. Eating fruits and vegetables, exercising in some form regularly, and finding time for relaxation, love, and gratitude are the simplest steps towards health.

The rest is just details.

Getting back to basics

Simple Health Action Steps

1. Today for a snack eat an apple with almond butter or peanut butter instead of a sugary candy bar or packaged snack food.

2. Eat dinner at the table with your family. Encourage everyone to stay there until every person has finished eating.

3. Read a little bit each day. Our local library reminds us that 20 minutes of reading is exercise for the brain. A free library membership is all you need to get in your mental workout.

4. Turn off the TV. Go outside, take a walk, plant some herbs, or get out a board game.

Chapter 6

Learn to Cook, and Make it Fun

When we first married, Dr. April was definitely the chef. My idea of cooking involved pre-mixed pancake batter that only required me to add water. While she prepared delicious cuisine using an array of spices that delighted the senses, most of what I made had to be covered in syrup.

Honestly, cooking intimidated me. I knew that some food was delicious (hers) while some food was not (mine). But I had no idea what made the difference. Then my amazing wife started showing me some things, teaching me about the spices, having me help her in the kitchen, and suddenly, I started getting it. Not only did I find myself able to prepare tasty meals, I found myself enjoying the process.

Today we cook all the time. Sometimes it's either one of us, sometimes we do it together. It has become something that we love to share with each other and enjoy the time (and health benefits) that it brings.

Let's first talk about a few of the health benefits you'll get from cooking at home. When we teach nutrition courses we always do an exercise where students evaluate the health of a meal found at a local restaurant. With nutrition information so easy to find these days, the students bring in the nutrition facts from pizza places, Mexican restaurants, sandwich shops, and fast food joints. They then go through choosing a meal they would typically order and identifying the amounts of calories, fat, sodium, sugars, etc. that would be in their meal. After calculating their results, they are always stunned by what they found.

Eating out typically leads to the realization that you reach almost your entire requirement of calories, sodium, sugar, and more in just one meal. Order a pizza and you get your quota of sodium for both today and tomorrow. Pick up some drive-thru and you may get more calories and fat in that one meal than you would have all day cooking at home. You would be amazed at just what is in the food that you get whenever you eat out. The experience for our students is always eye opening.

We recommend starting by, of course, keeping it simple. One of the first meals I learned to create was stir-fry. Why? Because I could take a bunch of vegetables (carrots, broccoli, celery, onion, mushroom, zucchini, etc.) cut them up and throw them in a pan with a little oil and soy sauce. I'd add a few spices like ginger and garlic, steam a pot of rice, and then mix it all together when it was done. It was easy, very basic, incredibly healthy, and surprisingly delicious.

By making this simple meal at home versus getting it at the local take-out we calculated that we reduced the calories by nearly half, the sodium by about 75%, nearly eliminated simple sugars, had far less fat, and at the same improved the nutrient content of the that meal significantly over our restaurant options. And we had a great time together!

We progressed to adding spinach and mushrooms to our eggs, finding out how to make pancakes from scratch, baking our own bread, and now Dr. April even makes Kombucha (a fermented drink) at home.

Here's a key on why it works so well for us and what is a must to make it work for you......it has to be FUN! Excitedly approach new recipes and foods like a kid looks at bugs outside. Turn on some music to dance to, pour a glass of wine, savor the aromas, have your family help you, and make it a good time. This is where cooking really became something I wanted to do and didn't feel obligated to do. Once you get the basic skills and knowledge you can start experimenting with new techniques, new recipes, or even substituting your own preferred foods in for others within a particular recipe. The possibilities become endless.

There are plenty of places you can go to learn some basic skills. Many career colleges offer evening classes showing you how to make a variety of dishes. Often you get to actually make the meal during class and try it right there providing immediate feedback. You can learn to cook Italian, Mediterranean, Chinese, Korean, and even how to grill. Now you can find the opportunity to do couples classes as well. It can make for a cool date night to do this. (Yes, you cook your own food but at least it's different than the old dinner and a movie and is far more interactive and collaborative.)

Learning to cook will drastically alter the basic ingredients that you feed your body. It may take some time, require you to endure a few failures, and then ask for creativity to make recipes healthier. But in the end, you feed your body well and it will thank you for it. By taking it another level and making it really fun, you'll feed your soul, too. It's your own brand of "soul food."

Learn to cook, make it fun

Simple Health Action Steps

1. Plan on making at least one meal at home this week using only fresh ingredients.

2. Find out what makes cooking fun for you. Do you need music to sing along with, a glass of wine to sip on, or enjoy the quiet time of creating something that serves you?

3. Experiment changing recipes to make them healthier. If you already cook, take your favorite recipe and see what you could substitute so it becomes a health food. Use some of the other recommendations in this book to guide you.

4. Teach your kids and let them help you. How much healthier would our kids be today and in the future if they knew how to prepare fresh, tasty meals for themselves?! And they'll know it can be fun! (not a chore to complain about or perform).

Chapter 7

Love - Express It, Share It, Receive It, and Feel Love

This is the first of our recommendations that steps outside the box of all the physical things you can do yourself and relies completely on your ability to work with thoughts and feelings. It's far more abstract and difficult to measure than eating an apple or drinking water in the morning. But the nature of this simple act regarding a deep emotion can change your entire life...always for the better.

In fact, the very morning that I'm writing this started off ugly. I woke up in a "bad mood," my body hurt, my thoughts were angry, and I knew that I was out of sorts with no real reason for any of it. Everything felt toxic, heavy, and irritated. Even my morning meditation didn't shake it off.

And in one moment it all began to melt away. April noticed something in me that wasn't quite right. She asked if I needed a hug, which she gracefully gave, and asked what was going on. Without even being able to fully describe the feelings that were burning me up, sharing even just a shred of what I was experiencing in the midst of her love took the edge off. I felt myself open up more and become deeply grateful for her embrace. Then in one beautiful moment, our little three year old came and turned our hug of two into an embrace of three. The softness of that moment was the perfect solution to the rough start of this day.

Through the release of certain hormones, love strengthens the immune system, relaxes the heart, soothes digestion, and provides mental clarity.

While this conversation around love may seem esoteric and maybe unfounded in regards to health, its implications are far from nonsense. Your body is largely built through your emotions under the guidance of a structure called your hypothalamus located deep in the central portion of your brain. Here, sadness or peace, anger or love are taken from a mental process to a physical reality as the hypothalamus begins a cascade of reactions that develop and circulate hormones around your body. In this sense you literally build your body based on the emotions you experience.

Positive emotions, especially one as powerful as love, heals the brain as well. Causing the release of neurotransmitters like dopamine and serotonin, love strengthens the immune system, relaxes the heart and blood vessels, soothes digestion, and provides clarity in thought[1]. The euphoric sensation you feel when experiencing deep love is profoundly healing for the entire body. That's why we feel so good when we are feeling love for another and feeling loved in return.

This concept has tremendous impact on the things you do that are designed to improve your health. We've known a number of people who do everything "right" in regards to their health. They eat salad constantly, regularly hit the gym, drink an ocean of water, and know everything there is to know about supplements that support their bodies. Yet they are miserable. They hate salad but eat it because they feel like they have to. The same old gym routine is stagnant and boring so they cover up the display on the treadmill hoping to just get through their arbitrary quota of minutes passes or miles pounded. And so it goes.

By going about health this way they unintentionally destroy it. They turn healthy habits into stressful tasks and activate breakdown mechanisms in the body instead of building it up and making it stronger. This is why you can't judge health based on body size or weight. Some skinny people appear physically healthy but are mentally and emotionally sick. While we've also known people who are little bit overweight or don't fit society's image of what health looks like and yet they are profoundly healthy living from a place of peace, gratitude, and love.

One major part of this experience that is difficult to describe with words on a page is the importance of you *feeling love*. Not just recognizing that you love your children or significant other. But allowing yourself to feel their love in you. To fully receive it and accept it - letting it wash over you. Experience the warmness in your chest, the flutter of your heart, the way blood flows throughout your body more easily. Notice and receive the blessing. Love is more than a thought process. It is a high sensory phenomenon that engages and activates every part of your being. It connects you to others as well as connects the physical/mental you to the soul part of you. When you really feel it, you completely alter the physiology of the body creating harmony, relaxation, and healing.

Love is felt in the moments. The in-between times and thoughts, when space is created for you to become aware of what is happening around you and within you. All you have to do is be open to it. Share love whenever, however you can and it will show itself to you. When it presents itself to you, accept it with open arms and allow yourself to feel it move through your chest, arms, stomach, and legs. It may take time to fully realize this step. Days, months, even years in some cases. Begin by being open to the idea, question its validity, experiment with the sensation, and see what happens for you.

We can't know exactly what your experience of love will be. But we do know that opening yourself to this profound transformative emotion changes everything.

Love – Express, Share, Receive, Feel

Simple Health Action Steps

1. Take a moment right now and think of something you love. Kids, spouse, nature, even chocolate! Notice where and how it feels in your body. Describe it to yourself and make a mental note of it. Is it warm? Relaxing? Exhilarating? Inspiring? Tingling? There is no wrong answer here. Just notice and accept.

2. With knowledge of what love feels like within you, find moments during your day where you can generate this feeling for yourself. While driving to work, making dinner, mowing the lawn, or sending emails see if you can create this feeling of love in your body just like you did in Action Step #1.

3. Do everything from a place of this love. If eating a salad is misery, find some other way to eat your veggies. Or at least another type of salad that you'll enjoy. Always make sure you are acting from this position of "I choose to" and not from "I have to." You can't force love.

Chapter 8

Mix Things Up and Keep it Fresh

One of the biggest challenges faced by nearly all of us is the onset of boredom. Every New Year's millions of people start working towards goals with excitement and enthusiasm. By mid-February it's estimated that well over half of everyone who set an initial intention has quit the pursuit. In fact, they now started calling certain Monday's in the first two months of the year "Blue Mondays" because it's a day of collective sadness where most people give up on our goals.

If you mix things up just a little bit you accomplish two things. One, you don't get bored and that keeps you moving forward. Two, the consistent shifts and changes that keeps things fresh is stimulation for your body and actually is a major mechanism that stimulates growth in the brain and the muscles. What can you do to continually add freshness to your life? Here's a few options we've been particularly fond of using for ourselves.

When it comes to exercise, variety really is the spice of life. We're both pretty lucky in that we enjoy spending time in a gym lifting weights or doing intense core exercises. Still, when we've done this as our ONLY routine for even just a couple weeks, it gets dull.....fast. So we always mix up the week with different exercises. Dr. April is a yoga instructor so yoga is a consistent practice for us. A few years ago we took up training with an instructor learning Muay Thai. The mixed martial art style of punches, kicks, a little grappling, and trying to dodge those same moves is exhilarating. The body loves this adding an aspect of speed not there in traditional weight lifting or yoga. The kicking, punching, and blocking activate different muscle groups in multiple sequences that stimulates their growth.

Your body responds well to change. In order to have continued success you have to mix things up and continually engage the mind and body

Maybe something like Muay Thai isn't for you. But Ju Jitsu may be, or regular boxing, or a dance class like Zumba, Pilates, or maybe a ballroom dance class. You see how fit those people are who go on Dancing with the Stars! Point is, engaging your body in a different way with fresh movements of the same muscles triggers their growth, metabolism, and health. Learning different exercises and applying them into my weekly (at least monthly) routines has been a major factor in preventing burnout.

What's cool is that this same process works for your mind. If you want to maintain mental clarity, high energy, and intellectual acuity both while going through your day at work and in the many years to come, you have to stimulate your brain like your muscles. In reality, exercise of the physical body is profoundly important for its ability to train your brain at the same time. That said, there are mental exercises or brain gymnastics that you can perform regularly to continually stimulate the mind and grow a healthy brain.

There are some different websites out there that provide great brain training programs. A number of apps are available for download on your phones that have a wide range of exercises designed to activate your mind. One we prefer to use is Lumosity[1]. They even have a free downloadable trial version. What you'll notice is that the games you play require paying attention to multiple things at the same time. You may have to find a miniscule difference among objects, switch tasks from identifying letters to numbers, remember a card you saw three cards back and determine if it matches the one you currently see, manage many things happening at the same time, and more. To top it off, nearly every one of them is timed. This is a healthy way of stressing the brain much like exercise stresses the muscles. You can continue to do this by filling out crosswords, doing Sudoku, reading books, taking classes on subjects you know little about, or even learning a new hobby.

But maybe the area that gets most boring is what we put in our mouths. Food, when well prepared with a flare that tingles the senses, is exciting. Left to repeat the same old thing time and time again with no sensational qualities, food becomes dull. Fast food companies know all about this effect. That is why they continually put out commercials trying to convince you that they are somehow different. They know that you just might get excited about a taco over another hamburger and fries. Or they take certain meals available for only limited times. It may even work once or twice.

But what continues to happen? They have to make grander versions of weird mixtures. Imagine a chalupa wrapped inside a taco filled with tamale on a bed of fried potatoes. Sounds bazaar, right? The only thing we find stranger than that concoction is how someone would actually eat it. But while this is a fictional food now similar creations are developed all the time.

Keeping variety in your food is crucial to your success with any new changes. If you've ever tried a diet that says you have to eat this certain food at this certain time for this predetermined amount of weeks you know what we mean. Most people drop their diet changes quicker than any others because it becomes bland. Eating a salad with a couple shreds of carrot and a slice of tomato every day is *really* boring. This boredom often leads to people quitting early with little or no results.

Continue to try new foods, learn to cook a new recipe, and find a way to not eat the same meals all the time. There are literally hundreds of thousands (probably more) of recipes out there on the internet just a few clicks away[2]. Give it a shot!

Food stagnation is real it's a rut we get stuck in too. You find something healthy, easy, and quick and next thing you know it becomes a multiple times a week sort of meal. When this happens we make a concerted effort to have something we haven't had in months. It might be a homemade hamburger, fish tacos, vegetable lasagna, or crepes. By switching up just one thing, it somehow opens up our palate to considering all the other options we know are out there. It's just a matter of breaking free from the mundane and getting the excitement back into the show!

Mix things up and keep it fresh

Simple Health Action Steps

1. Vary your exercise routine to include many types of exercise each week. A typical, great week of workouts for us includes 3 days of weights, 1-2 days of yoga, and an intense day of Muay Thai

2. Keep a healthy mind that resists memory loss, dementia, and lack of sharpness by stimulating the mind with puzzles, books, and games that challenge you.

3. Create a binder of recipes for yourself so that when you get stuck in a food rut, you have a number of options at your immediate disposal to pick up and break free.

4. Remember that your muscles, brain, gut, and every other part of you is stimulated to grow and heal when you keep things fresh and mix it up.

Chapter 9

Addition Before Subtraction

One of the primary ways we are told to make positive changes and achieve goals is to get rid of those things that hold us back. Diets tell you to immediately quit this food, new fad workouts tell you to stop running, or maybe you're supposed to quit smoking cold turkey. While none of these pieces of advice may be bad per se, a large part of the reason people fail is because it's focused on what you take away. Shifting your focus on what you can ADD has shown to be an incredible tool in making positive changes.

It seems to work on a few levels, but here's why we have found such success within our own lives and those of our clients. Just eliminating something from your life often involves pain. Having relationships end hurts. Losing a business is painful. Not getting to have a full pot of coffee or your lunch time cigarette comes with the pain of withdrawals. No matter the situation, immediately losing something feels like a part of you is gone. Rationalizing it only goes so far. If part of you is missing (and that's honestly what it feels like when we give up something that was an integral part of our day) there's a void. A deep empty space begging to be filled.

Unfortunately, we usually fill it with something less than ideal. This is why many smokers who quit have a tendency to gain weight. They fill their void with food and have another challenge to deal with as the outcome. Similarly, sodas get replaced by sugary juices just as bad for you. Fried food is replaced by salty food. Television gets replaced by cell phones. This tendency shows up in nearly all aspects of our lives.

That's why we flip this process around and work on *adding* something in before *taking* something away. We prevent creating a void that needs to be filled and instead add a healthy trait or practice into an otherwise full day. The response is that people get to feel more fulfilled. They feel more alive and less like part of them is dying.

You can do this by choosing something, anything, to add into your day that would be beneficial to your health. Choose any one of the 20 other simple tips and apply it immediately. Don't deny yourself something that you treasure. But add in a tall glass of water in the morning. Go for a walk with your family in the evening before you turn on the TV. Put more spices in your home-cooked meal or tell someone "I love you."

Like love, what you'll find is that by giving you will receive. Giving yourself something to be proud of, like adding spinach to your eggs, builds the self-esteem and confidence to continue to add more healthy habits and make bigger changes. You'll feel the difference, recognize the changes, and then be propelled into doing more for yourself.

Eventually, you begin adding so much positive into your day that the negatives start to randomly disappear. You fill your day with all the things that make you feel energized, vibrant, and alive. Suddenly, there's no room for the things that don't serve your new energy level. It seems to simply vanish before your eyes. Not as something that required a crowbar to wrench out of your life, but something that you could release and willingly let go of because when you ate that food, had that thought, or skipped that workout, you felt worse than when you did the highest of all those actions.

This is the method we used for getting soda out of our regular habits. Growing up we both drank soda in our respective homes quite regularly. Kicking the habit cold turkey was tough. We craved the fizzy little bubbles and sweetness. Water felt boring after a couple days and if it was especially hot outside, ice cold water just didn't cut it. So instead of just dumping soda in one shot, we just kept adding water. Each sip of soda was accompanied by a sip of water. Besides it making us have to use the bathroom a lot, the process worked. Gradually we noticed that we felt better with higher water intake than we did with the soda. Our energy levels were better, skin cleared, sleep improved, and more. Next thing we knew, having a soda was shockingly sweet.

So sweet, in fact, that we could hardly drink it. Even today on the rare occasion we do have a soda, the two of us will split a 12oz. can.

We've seen this process work for many people. The psychological effect is worth noting and is important. But we've always been surprised at how much it seems to take the pressure off. Saying you're going on a diet often means giving up lunch with friends, drinks with the guys, or your Friday night pizza. Adding all the positives into your day has an almost reverse-psychology effect in helping you overcome bad habits.

If we were to recommend the "best" additions you could make that are simple, yet extremely effective they would go like this: Drink water first thing in the morning, add in a probiotic or fermented food, breathe deeply, and add at least one new food into your meals (spinach into eggs, cinnamon into cookies, etc.). You can choose any, but these are some that are so simple you can't go wrong and yet they do seem to have the impact you're looking for.

Just like we're taught in school, addition should come before subtraction.

Addition before subtraction

Simple Health Action Steps

1. Focus on *adding in healthy actions* **before** *eliminating negative habits.*

2. Choose one positive addition you can make to your day and add it today. It might just be going and getting a giant glass of water right now.

3. Add in another positive change in a week. Do it again the following week. Then see if you can begin a snowball of change where positive additions become easier and easier.

4. Allow your additions to begin replacing your negative habits. Kick the artificial sweeteners, use less salt, let go of soda, put down the cell phone at dinner, etc. You got this!

Chapter 10

Sweet Agony:
Avoid Artificial Sweeteners

There is seemingly nowhere that artificial sweeteners aren't found now. And that is dangerous. These super-sweet lab generated "sugars" have a number of neurological and physical concerns associated with them. With their widespread use it's also become extremely important to pay special attention to everything you buy and search the ingredient list for hidden artificial sweeteners.

First, let's look at why we recommend avoiding them like the plague. In the book *Excitotoxins*[1], Dr. Michael Blaylock outlines how artificial sweeteners (like MSG) affect the body. He explains that artificial sweeteners are a form of neurochemical that cause the brain to get overly excited. Undergoing the stress of this continual hyper activity, the cells of the brain actually start to die! Yes, the cells that help you walk, talk, think, speak, and breathe are put under extreme strain to the point of facing death. Which is why they are known as excito-*toxins*.

Think of it working like this. When you give a little kid a mountain of sugar you know what's going to happen. The child will get hyper, most likely be obnoxious and act out. But wait just 30 minutes and what comes next? The crash. They get tired, cranky, and lethargic. This is very similar to what happens with your neurons (brain cells). Except that your neurons could potentially face the death penalty.

Keeping that in mind, here's a small list of conditions, symptoms, and diseases that are linked with the use of artificial sweeteners: headaches, depression, dizziness, seizures, memory loss, diarrhea, weight gain, and possibly even Alzheimer's disease[2,3]. The way the body breaks down aspartame, the product used in Nutrasweet and Equal, it creates chemicals linked to cancer. Yes, that's right. There is a chemical process by which this food in your body can potentially lead to cancer![3] Doesn't sound so sweet any more does it.

Of course, what's the number one reason people use artificial sweeteners? Weight loss. Which makes this bit really depressing. *Use of artificial sweeteners have been linked to people gaining weight instead of losing it.* Their intention to shed a few pounds by eliminating sugar and using the no calorie fake stuff works exactly opposite than we would think. Instead, your body is "tricked" into actually holding onto more weigh, and storing it as dangerous fat around your organs[4].

Knowing now that these things are scary, it's important to know how to find them. As we said, they are everywhere hiding in many places you'd never expect to see them.

Our first realization with this came when we were buying coffee creamer. We both enjoyed the sweet flavor of hazelnut coffee creamer. It was sweet and rich and made us feel like we got a morning treat. Learning to read labels we were shocked to find that Splenda had made its way into our favorite creamer. Next we found it in nearly every yogurt and even in some forms of milk. We couldn't believe they had put this stuff in milk!

That led to more research and deeper scrutiny of everything. Suddenly, we realized these health-destroying neurochemicals were in foods we never would have imagined. It's a challenge find yogurt or cereal without it, our coffee creamer was gone (now we use heavy whipping cream), and flavored potato chips contain it, popular brands of gum use it, we even found it in vitamin supplements! Vitamins!!!

It really came down to this…if it says "Zero Calorie" or "No Sugar" you can bet it will have artificial sweeteners. This means diet sodas, low calorie/no calorie cookies and other desserts, fruit snacks, sports drinks, and any other products carrying claims like this are almost certain to contain excitotoxins. *You have to be diligent and read the labels of everything.* Even the products you can't possibly imagine containing artificial sweeteners like coffee creamer or cereal.

Without getting all conspiracy theory on you, it must be said that somehow our regulatory agencies like the FDA continue to allow companies to find new names and ways of hiding their use of the artificial sweeteners. This makes finding these things pretty hard to do at times. They give them names that sound like the real thing, like it comes from nature. Most even advertise themselves as slightly altered but better forms of real sugar.

You probably are well aware of the main three things to look out for, those commonly seen pink, blue, and yellow packets. You also may remember in the reading labels section to search for the word "artificial" as an easy marker to spot them. But there are a number of other potential names that food manufacturers are allowed to use that hide the sweeteners from simple identification.

Beware of these other names for artificial sweeteners: Saccharin (Equal), Sucralose (Splenda), Acesulfame K, Aspartame (NutraSweet), Neotame (new form of Aspartame), and the new kid on the block Amino Sweet.

One of the main complaints we get when presenting this topic is that regular sugar doesn't taste sweet enough anymore. People felt they *had* to have the fake stuff. It's because these artificial sweeteners trigger addictive receptors in your brain. They basically rewrite your code for what "sweet" is and now actual sugar isn't sweet. That's pretty messed up.

If you are trying to limit your actual sugar intake, we recommend a few other options to add into your diet. We still use sugar in our house. When we use it, it's the raw, cane sugar known as turbinado. We always work to get things in their most natural form. Outside of regular sugar try these natural substitutes: Stevia, Xylitol, Honey, Brown Rice Syrup, and Dextrose.

Avoid artificial sweeteners

Simple Health Action Steps

1. Go through your pantry and fridge to see if you find any foods that have artificial sweeteners in them. If so, dispose of them immediately.

2. Play a game at the grocery store and see if you can find foods that DON'T have artificial sweeteners. Remember to look for all the possible names. More detailed lists can be found online.

3. In the case you are diabetic, please check with your doctor before making any changes. But be sure to discuss this with them and seek out other professional opinions to make the best choice for you. As we often say, a diabetic shouldn't be choosing between regular soda and diet soda....they shouldn't be choosing soda at all.

Chapter 11

Taste Nature's Rainbow

Go to the produce area of the grocery store and you'll notice a beautiful sight. The variety of fruits and vegetables presents a rainbow of colors that is both appealing to the eye and pleasing to your body. Eating foods throughout the color spectrum provides a variety of different nutrients. The color of the fruit or vegetable is often indicative of what types of vitamins, minerals, and other healthy nutrients are found in that food. Consuming all the different colors assures that you will be providing your body a wide range of nutrients to heal and grow.

Look at these examples. Carrots are known for their health properties related to our eyes. Their orange color is an indication of the presence of Beta – Carotene which is important in the health and maintenance of our eyesight. Knowing that the red/orange color is linked to beta carotene and in turn our eyes, we can associate this health benefit to other orange foods including sweet potatoes and mangos[1,2].

Leafy green vegetables like spinach, romaine lettuce, and kale are known for having high levels of vitamin K and fiber[1,2]. We know that vitamin K helps form blood clots, and fiber is important for digestive health. Citrus fruit like lemons and limes are recognized for their high vitamin C content. We use vitamin C to heal wounds, fight infections, and take care of our skin.

A variety of colors reflects a variety of nutrients. Eat many different colors to provide your body all the various nutrients it needs to heal, recover and grow.

Dark, rich colored fruits indicate high levels of antioxidants. Blueberries, blackberries, raspberries, cherries, apples, and pears with beautifully deep colors use their mega-sized antioxidant levels to fight off inflammation and free radicals that can lead to cancer[1,2].

As you can see, eating a variety of color is important in our diets. It provides a full spectrum of flavors and nutrients to support our bodies in every function. From blood to eyes, immunity to digestive health, colors serve as a helpful tool for giving your body all the various nutrients it needs.

The other benefit is that color makes food look considerably more appetizing. We conducted a little experiment with some of our students to put this to the test. We put up pictures of four meals and asked which looks the most appealing. One meal was fried chicken with mashed potatoes and gravy. Another was a steak with a side of French fries and broccoli. The final two were both salads. One was a salad from a bag that had iceberg lettuce with a few strings of carrot and cabbage. The other was a lush green salad with spinach and romaine lettuce, carrots, red cabbage, walnuts, cucumber, mandarin orange and a piece of salmon. Everyone agreed that the salad with all the different bright, lush colors was the most appealing meal. And now you know it's also the most nutritious!

Marketers know this response. We had the chance to speak with a woman whose career was preparing food from popular companies for pictures and videos that would be used for commercials and ads. She showed us her "toolkit" of tweezers, clippers, brushes, and so on. The number of tools she had for making fake food look real and appetizing was amazing. It seemed like it would put most women's make-up kits to shame. That's why you see a picture for a burger on a commercial and it's layered with crisp lettuce, vibrant red tomato, perfectly round pickle, and delicately melted cheese. Then when you pick it up at the restaurant you get a floppy, dull, unappetizing mess.

We're drawn to color because of what it signifies to us...nutrients. It's your body's way of saying, "I would love some fiber, vitamin K, vitamin C, antioxidants, and beta carotene." Go eat that food!

You can create this for yourself at home using similar techniques. Just get a number of different colored vegetables and fruits and put them together. We make vibrant stir-fry using cabbage, carrots, broccoli, and yellow peppers. We add blueberries, strawberries, mango, pineapple, and kale or spinach to smoothies. Mixing reds, greens, yellows, purples, and oranges really stimulates your appetite. It also provides a load of nutrients for everything your body needs.

Taste nature's rainbow

Simple Health Action Steps

1. With each meal, try to have three (3) different colors on your plate.

2. Mix up the different colors you eat together for a full profile of nutrients in various combinations. This is both stimulating for your body and for your taste buds and helps prevent boredom.

Chapter 12

Practice Forgiveness for Yourself

So you ate that donut at the office. Now you feel guilty. You had been doing so well and were so excited about your plan towards health. Suddenly, it seems your weaknesses have been revealed and you are doomed. Just another example of why it won't work for you, right?

Not so fast! Ok, you had the donut or (insert your proverbial donut here). Perhaps you missed your workout three days this week. Or you spent all day yesterday totally angry. So what? Sure, it may not have been your best choice for the path you've chosen. But it doesn't mean you've gotten so far off track that you can't get back. This is a time for learning and for forgiveness.

We all have times when situations find us choosing from options that we otherwise might not make. It is important to remember that one small deviation doesn't ruin an entire plan. If you feel bad about your choice, show yourself some grace and forgive your misstep. Then get right back to doing what you had set your intention to do. Often you'll find you haven't lost the momentum you had at all.

> *It's important to remember that one small deviation doesn't ruin a whole plan. Just pick up where you left off and keep going.*

A common place we find ourselves facing this scenario is when we travel. Whether we're heading out of town to speak somewhere, attend a conference, or visit family, following the normal health routine is more challenging. Airports aren't known for their health food, hotel beds are less comfortable and familiar, and there's stress just not being in your regular flow. With all that happening, it's real easy to get upset about how far off course you may find yourself.

The issue is that many people let this one event completely ruin their progress. We seem to believe that one moment outside of the plan spells disaster. People beat themselves up over being angry, going to bed late, or not meditating. All of which defeats the intention behind doing them in the first place. Instead, we should choose to forgive ourselves. Nothing goes exactly as planned for anyone. It's not a matter of imperfection, it's a matter of life. Show yourself a little grace and continue right where you left off. Your progress isn't voided by a few down days. You don't have to start over. Just simply pick up where you were and continue from there.

Here is an important rule to live by. If you're going to eat not-on-your-plan foods, or have drinks with friends, or feel like staying in and watching a movie, do it! The key is to not feel guilty about it. For example, we love pizza and red wine. Once or twice a month we get a pizza and a bottle of wine to enjoy. And during that time, we don't express one ounce of remorse. We revel in the delight of our choice. But the next day, we're right back to our normal plans.

Remember: Life is supposed to be *fun!*

Practice forgiveness for yourself

Simple Health Action Steps

1. When you find yourself in a situation where you haven't stayed on course with your goals, pause for a moment, take a deep breath, and say "I completely love and forgive myself."

2. While you're eating that pizza or skipping that Zumba class, love every second of it! Then pick up where you left off tomorrow.

Chapter 13

Practice Forgiveness for Others

Certainly you knew this was coming. While we have a tendency to be extremely hard on ourselves, few things in life are as toxic as holding onto grudges or upsets related to other people. Friends, family, acquaintances and perfect strangers run roughshod through our minds causing distress and leading to stress. Forgiving those who you feel have wronged you is one of the most soothing practices you can employ.

Here's a practice for you to follow adapted from teachers including Dr. Sue Morter and Rev. Dr. Michael Beckwith.[1,2] It should be noted that your ability to forgive another has nothing to do with them forgiving you. Actually, the practice I'm going to share with you is one that I've been walked through by other healers to work through my own upsets and patterns that continually cause me grief and heartache. What I also like about it is that the person or event that you're forgiving doesn't need to be present. If John punched you in the face in high school you don't need to call up John or skype with him to let it go. Forgiveness is a very personal event and feeling. You can work with this completely on your own and no one else ever has to know.

NOTE: Some events and people may cause deep emotional upset. While you first use this practice, it is *highly* recommended that you choose a person or event that won't trigger major reactions. In other words, it may not be best to work on forgiving someone who abused you as a child on your first attempt with this practice. It may be far more beneficial to forgive someone who spilled your coffee or took your parking spot.

Sit comfortably resting your hands on your lap or folded softly in front of you. Take a couple deep breaths to calm the mind. Recall a situation or person who upset you in some way. See their face, recall the circumstances, picture them sitting right in front of you. Notice what you feel as you see this person. You may be mildly irritated or 100% pissed off. Either way, take two more deep breaths. Now looking at this person simply say to them, "I forgive you." You may feel like saying it two or three times. Perhaps you'll repeat it in a slow, personal mantra for a couple minutes. See if the feeling of upset in your body is lessening. Have you backed off from 100% rage to 50%? Can you maybe just look at the person and not feel so outraged?

Once you've noticed the initial emotion being reduced, picture the person turning around and walking away. Know that the situation has been resolved as long as you're willing to fully let it go. If it pops up again, just repeat the process. *It's not failure, but recognition of how our brain patterns sometimes need repeated input to change their circuitry.*

As simple as this practice is, we can attest to having experienced the benefits. Being married often means having disagreements. Arguments over money, kids, groceries, and other responsibilities just happen. Hanging on to small upsets starts a snowball of stress. Most people have probably been caught in the middle of an undone chore turning into a list of wrongdoing. Recognizing that mindset and taking even a second to allow forgiveness has been crucial to our happy marriage.

Forgiveness can happen in an instant or feel like it takes forever. Some emotions and events have many layers you'll need to run through before reaching real full forgiveness. You can try adding in other modalities like Tapping, neurolinguistic programming, or EMDR[3] to aid in the process. But we recommend if using other modalities to have someone qualified in those practices to assist you. Allowing yourself the opportunity to heal these open wounds is truly one of the more powerful tools to radically change your health and your life.

Practice forgiveness for others

Simple Health Action Step

1. Pick one person today and use this technique. Maybe you'll do this 5 times with just this one person today. Work through it until you feel the charge of that person decline to nearly nothing. Repeat as you need with other people and events that cause upset.

Chapter 14

Disconnect from Tech:
Even a Few Minutes Helps

Take a quick quiz. How many times a day do you check your email? How many phone calls do you make in a day? Do you constantly check your cell phone for messages or missed calls even after you get home from work? Do you prefer to talk to friends and family by text message instead of actually talking to them? Are you always making sure your phone is nearby? How many times during the day do you mindlessly scroll through Facebook, Pinterest, Twitter, or TV channels not even really paying attention but acting out of boredom or habit?

If we are being perfectly honest I think most of us would be somewhat amazed at our answers to these questions. There is little doubt that we have become a society not only reliant on technology but absorbed by it. Frequently we judge someone's popularity by the number of twitter followers they have or look for satisfaction by having the latest smartphone. Interestingly enough, it seems that the more our phones do, the less they are used as actual phones.

Having technology is wonderful and I benefit from it as much as anyone else does. However, being totally connected all the time leaves us little time to authentically share and connect with those around us. And more importantly, little time to relax, unwind, and take care of ourselves.

Constantly scrolling through social media or playing games has a number of effects on us. Often we delay going to sleep, drinking water, cooking that healthy dinner, spending time with family, reading a book, or taking time to meditate or pray. Fortunately, as with almost everything, there are very simple things you can do to squash this habit.

We often recommend creating a space in your home or particular times of the day where there is a complete disconnection from your technological gadgets. Make a "NO PHONE ZONE" or whatever you want to call it. Spend just a few minutes there a day either when you wake up, when you get home, right before bed or whenever works for you. Some of the times we've found working best for our family is early morning when we tend to read and during dinner time when we can all sit together. And although we haven't made this an official house rule (we may be getting close with a three year old who already understands more about these gadgets than we do), the intention of those times is clear and we hold to them.

The benefits of this simple time, maybe even ten or fifteen minutes at a time, is profound. You'll go to bed and actually fall asleep, your children will get more attention and you'll create better relationships, thoughts and inspirations will run through you, and stress levels drop.

We bet you will be surprised at just how rejuvenating it can be to simply have quiet, relaxing time to yourself. Your stress will decrease. Your joy will increase. And you will have a sense of being refreshed from the inside-out. We recently saw a family at our office after they returned from taking their daughter on a cruise for her graduation gift. Interestingly, of all the things they saw and did, each said one of the best parts of the trip was taking a four day break from texts, calls, and social media.

When low on energy, disconnecting from technology can be one of the most rejuvenating things you can do.

However, be aware that this time can also be rather revealing. If during that time you notice yourself anxiously worried about missed calls or the latest gossip, then your sense of attachment is gaining control of you. Teachers see this with students every day. In the middle of class, we see them sending text messages or checking email. The desire to be connected is so consuming they allow their world to revolve around Facebook and twitter posts and neglect the reason for being where they are sitting. They often then wonder why their grades are so poor or why the teacher has to make the course so hard.

Does that sound like you? Do you ever wonder why you never seem to get anything done but spend a couple hours in front of the TV every night? Or do you go to dinner as a family and look around the table to see everyone staring at phones and ignoring each other?

Please know we are not comparing technology to the dark evils of fiction novels. Quite the contrary. We love technology and have our favorite shows to watch along with games on our cell phones. That also means we know how easy it is to slip into a habit of spending more time focused on the technology than on other people, even ourselves.

We've ditched our cable a number of times. And each time we do something peculiar happens. We read more. We talk more. We play more. We cook more. We walk and exercise more. We meditate more. We even have sex more! It seems that the less time we spend with technology the more of everything else we really desire in life is there.

This is easy, but it takes some discipline. Our society's attachment to technology is strong. You may realize just how much you get sucked into to the digital fortress. Give your family and yourself the time and peace you deserve by spending a little bit of time every day taking a break from technology and putting your attention on them.

Disconnect from technology

Simple Health Action Steps

1. Create time each day to disconnect from the "world." Make a room in your home a No Phone Zone. This is a great idea for the bedroom especially.

2. Pay attention to how much other parts of your life change with this practice. Do you get more done or spend more time with your family? Is your energy higher and do you feel better?

Chapter 15

Straighten Up! See a Chiropractor

Chiropractors have become very popular for their ability to relieve low back and neck pain, sciatica, headaches and many other conditions. It used to be that people sought out chiropractors as a last ditch effort to avoid surgery or because they've tried everything else and found little to no help. That perception is changing, and with it people are recognizing how truly beneficial seeing a chiropractor can be.

Chiropractic is a system of analyzing and realigning joints in the body to allow the body to work at its highest level. It deals primarily with the spine because the spine has a very powerful connection to the master system of the body, the nervous system. *By correcting misalignments in the body that cause tension and inflammation, adjustments allow a relaxation of the tight muscles and irritated nerves that cause pain, stiffness, numbness, tingling, or muscle spasms.* Because it works directly with the nervous system, it also provides benefits to the entire body. This is why people have gone in to see chiropractors for back pain and noticed improvements in digestion, circulation, sleep, and even vision.

And there's more. Regular visits to a chiropractor have shown to be an effective means of maintaining health, superior to other treatments for back pain and in the long run even saving you significant amounts of money[1]. One study found that it could save you over $1,000 per person every two years[2]! That can lead to a pretty nice vacation!

But the real benefits come from living day to day feeling loose, active, healthy, and energetic. Many people who consistently see a chiropractor don't need to point to areas of pain or discomfort because they don't have them. Imagine how great it would be to walk around *without* achy joints or sore muscles and have the full unlimited physical ability to do all the things you love to do. Imagine being able to work in the garden, go for a run, ski huge mountains, and play outside with your grandkids free of aches and pains. Chiropractic can help get you there.

Why is it necessary to see a chiropractor in the first place? Because generally our lifestyles have a way of leading to those misalignments that irritate nerves and muscles. We sit at computers, in our cars, or on the couch for hours every day. Usually we do all this sitting with bad posture staring at screens and slouching. Accidents, slips, falls, or even an intense or new workout can wrench things out of place. If left out of place for long periods, the body develops muscle memory of this misaligned and irritating position. Now you almost constantly suffer from smoldering, annoying pain. And while you can do a great deal to cure these ills with other practices, it is nearly impossible to correct these misalignments by yourself.

This also doesn't have to be something you use only when you're hurting. People who continue to see a chiropractor (even after their pain is gone) realize how great they feel and simply want to stay that way. They play, live, work and do all the same things everyone else is doing. However, when they notice they don't feel quite right they make a point to visit to their chiropractor. Instead a minor tweak turning into a festering ache, it's resolved immediately and they go right back to living as they were.

As a husband-wife chiropractic team we're lucky to have this service available whenever we want it. Today we still adjust each other about every two weeks to keep our bodies healthy and strong. Research suggests we all should get adjusted at least every three weeks since scar tissue leading to arthritis can develop in that short amount of time. Chiropractic adjustments remove the scar tissue and may be prevent long term arthritis and breakdown of the spine.

Are there different types of chiropractors and the way they practice? Absolutely. But all work to realign the joints and provide smooth, healthy action of the nerves, muscles, and other systems of the body. It is very safe, extremely cost-effective, and incredibly beneficial to your health.

Visit a Chiropractor

Simple Health Action Step

1. Schedule a visit with a local chiropractor and see how they can help you reach maximum health.

Chapter 16

Eat Fermented Foods

Fermentation is one of the oldest forms of preserving foods. It is also one of our best methods for being happy, healthy, and emotionally well. You may have heard of probiotics, which are commonly found in the form of supplements. If you have stayed plugged into this world of probiotics, you may have begun to hear that now you also need to take *pre*biotics. Sometimes, it may feel like a never ending list of pills to take. The good news is, when you consume a variety of fermented, or cultured, foods you are getting more probiotics and prebiotics than you could ever consume in a supplement.

What are prebiotics and probiotics? Prebiotics are the foods that the probiotics eat and then utilize in order to produce wonderful benefits for your body. Probiotics are microorganisms like bacteria that live in and on our bodies forming what science calls our *microbiome.*

When we have a nice variety of microbes growing in our colon we are able to keep harmful bacteria and fungi from creating disease in the body. When the number of potentially disease-causing (pathogenic) microbes populate the body in higher amounts than the helpful and healing ones it is called dysbiosis. Dysbiosis affects many different parts and systems of the body. While no two people exhibit the exact same symptoms, some signs include *food intolerance, indigestion or irritable bowel, headaches and migraines, ADD/ADHD and other behavior disorders, rashes, autoimmune diseases or even depression*[1].

> ***80% of your immune system and serotonin are produced in your gut.***

How does dysbiosis occur? What you put into your body is the primary cause. Processed, chemical and sugar laden foods create an environment that allows potentially pathogenic microbes to thrive, while slowly killing the beneficial microbes. Medications like antibiotics don't play favorites in their hunt for bacteria, viruses, or fungi. They kill without remorse which means they take out the good guys as much as the bad. Combine that with a sedentary lifestyle where the intestines aren't stimulated to move and you in effect create a toxic dump filled with dead and decaying waste. Yes, it's as gross as it sounds.

So what are some of the major benefits of bringing healthy microbes into the system? Eighty percent of your immune system is in your intestines. These organisms aid in the immune function by fighting pathogenic microbes, forming antibodies against pathogens, and chelating or detoxifying heavy metals and toxins that our system can't handle. They help balance the production of stomach acid and produce a variety of essential vitamins for our body, like vitamin K2, niacin, folic acid and more. Eighty percent of your serotonin, the "happy hormone" is produced or found in your gut[2]. This hormone is a precursor to many hormones, including melatonin, the "sleep hormone". The added benefit of weight loss and weight management are just another reason to eat or drink fermented foods.

There are a variety of ways that you can get these microbes into your vibrant living plan. You can supplement with pills. However, our experience tells us you won't feel the full benefits because it will be limited on sheer number of microbes you'll consume and the variety of different microbes present will be smaller compared to eating fermented foods. That said, for those that are extremely depleted of intestinal microbes, it is a good option to take probiotics in supplement form for a while and start adding fermented foods in slowly to help replenish the system.

If eating bacteria willingly through supplements or foods sounds strange or weird, we think you'll agree it sounds less awkward than being the recipient of a poop transplant! Yes, this is a real thing. When people have taken so many rounds of antibiotics that it has destroyed their normal microbiome, they often suffer from many health problems some of which can be life-threatening. For a speedy recovery, there is a trend of supplying fecal transplants into the intestines to aid in colonizing new bacteria[3]. So there's that option.

Or you can simply eat a variety of fermented/cultured foods every day. Fermented foods include sauerkraut, kimchi, pickles, kombucha, kefir, or many other pickled vegetables. You can make them at home or buy them in the store. Truly fermented foods have live cultures and should only be found in the refrigerated section of the store. If it's not refrigerated, probably best not to buy it. And as always, read the label and make sure there are no added ingredients like food coloring, sweeteners, or preservatives (the bacteria do that for you).

Sometimes people will experience a detox effect, where symptoms may briefly worsen or constipation may occur, when they start with fermented foods. This is usually the system righting itself by trying to eliminate that toxic dump and flushing out the cells. It is better to begin with adding small amounts (2-4 oz.) once a day and then increase to small amounts with every meal. This should help the body handle the change with more ease. Drinking more water and going for walks will help move things along with more efficiency.

It took us awhile to really understand the benefit of fermented foods. Today we use a Perfect Pickler to make homemade goods that top nachos and go in smoothies. And we really enjoy the benefits.

Eat fermented foods

Simple Health Action Step:

1. Start slow. Add kefir or kombucha to your morning breakfast, but less than a quarter of a cup. After a couple of days, add sauerkraut or kimchi to your lunch, again keeping it at under a quarter cup. Once you feel yourself balancing and feeling more energized, start adding more to each meal.

2. Variety is the key. By consuming a variety of cultured foods you will consume a large diversity of microbes. Try different foods with each meal.

3. Learn to make your own. You don't need a lot of fancy equipment to ferment your favorite vegetables. An easy way to get started is with the Perfect Pickler, which can be found on Amazon.com.

Chapter 17

Maximum Serenity, Maximum Sleep

We were recently in Omaha speaking at a health conference and it provided ample opportunity to speak with people about a number of topics. One that came up then, and continues to be a major concern, is sleep. Talking with people from teenagers to folks in their 80s it is very apparent that people have trouble with sleep and suffer a number of effects because of it.

We spoke to the parents of one teenager who had even seen their honor roll student suffer sleep deprivation to such a degree she was regressing to a point of having difficulty reading or even speaking clearly. Their outgoing, active daughter was becoming withdrawn and not participating in her favorite school activities. She was tested for every disorder they could think of. But the only real problem anyone could find was her inability to get consistent, restful, rejuvenating sleep.

Sleep is when our brain processes the day, transfers short term memory into long term memory, and runs through subconscious protocols providing understanding and meaning. If you couldn't tell from the story of the regressing honor roll student, sleep is a big deal!

As a whole, our country is sleep deprived. Whether it is not getting enough hours of sleep (7-9), or getting poor quality sleep, the fact remains that most of us our tired. There are some very simple things anyone can do to improve their sleep. Among the most critical are creating a peaceful space that aids in sleep and using techniques that relax and clam the mind.

A major key to making a peaceful, restful place is to make it very dark. The darker your bedroom is the better you will sleep. This is based on the function of a gland in your body called the Pineal gland. The pineal gland reacts to light to determine how much of a hormone called Melatonin to release.

When a room is very bright, like a classroom, office building, or smartphone screen, very little melatonin is released and you tend to stay awake. With increasing darkness, more melatonin circulates through the brain. The bump in melatonin levels aids the body in sleep by slowing everything down and putting the body into a restful state.

Take out televisions, put up blackout curtains, leave cell phones in other rooms, and do whatever you need to make your room as dark as absolutely possible. We go so far as to cover the face of our alarm clocks so the bright LED lights don't create an undesired brightness. Whatever steps you want to take, do them tonight and start noticing the difference it creates.

In regards to relaxing and calming the mind, one of the best practices is deep breathing. As mentioned in an earlier section, deep breathing changes the physiology of the body from a stressful state to a restful one. Breathing for long counts (an inhale of 7, hold for 4, and exhale for 10) drastically slows the mind and calms the body.

Many people with regular sleep problems get stressed out about falling asleep. Then suddenly they're stressed out about being stressed out about not being able to sleep! It's like those times when you wake up at 3 a.m. and can't fall back asleep all the while wondering how you'll get through the day if you don't fall back asleep. So you toss and turn putting pressure on yourself to fall back asleep. Even during this time, deep breathing is the most beneficial practice for you to use. It's worked great for us in these exact circumstances.

Here's one other tool we use to help create restful sleep: reduce the exposure to any kind of distractions or major stimulation in the 15 minutes right before bed. In the moments where you are preparing to for bed each night, make it as relaxing as possible. It's a perfect time for reading (an actual book, not a kindle or tablet). With softer lighting you release more melatonin and while reading engages the mind it doesn't provide stimulation in the way that electronics do. Give yourself a fifteen minute window before bed where you turn off all the electronics. Go through your nightly routine of brushing your teeth, having a small glass of water, reading, or maybe journaling.

Making this a regular habit becomes a way of you letting your body know that it's time for bed and allows it to prepare for rest. It triggers the mind to quiet, the muscles to relax, and gets you in a state ready for sleep.

Then, turn off the lights creating a dark room allowing melatonin to be released at higher levels. Give gratitude for the day while practicing deep breathing and instead of counting sheep count your blessings. If any stressful or negative thoughts do arise, honor them and gently shift your mind back to your breathing practice and thoughts of thankfulness.

Repeated over time, developing neural patterns that support this process and lead to rest, you can get back to having deep, restful sleep that rejuvenates the mind, re-energizes the body, and builds optimism for living. Your results will be so valuable you will be motivated take on life's challenges and start taking control of your life at every level.

Maximum sleep

Simple Health Action Steps

1. Make your room as dark as possible. Remove anything that glows or emits some form of ambient light. This will boost your melatonin and allow for deeper sleep.

2. Practice a deep breathing exercise inhaling for a slow count of seven, hold for four, and exhale for a count of 10.

3. Create a routine for the 15 minutes before bed where electronics are turned off, you go through your nightly preparations, and spend the last few minutes in soft light and deep silence.

Chapter 18

Meditate, Pray, Relax

When it comes to instilling and maintaining health, most everything is based around "doing" something. Interestingly, one of the practices that has brought us the biggest benefit is what some would refer to as the practice of "being." Being in meditation, prayer, and through them relaxation, is as essential to true health transformation as is any single action you can take.

While both meditation and prayer can be taken to deep spiritual levels of connectedness, and through that deep healing, on a more simple level they both promote deep relaxation. Sitting in a certain position turning your focus inward accesses a calmness that you can find in every breath. This relaxes the mind and the body which impacts the physiology that runs your organs and cells.

Relaxation helps to turn off the "fight or flight" response and puts the body into a far more efficient mode as discussed in the section on breathing. It lowers the release of the hormone cortisol and in turn soothes the cells allowing them to create more energy while producing less acidic waste. This in turn heals the body at every level and provides a rejuvenating flush of energy to the entire body[1].

These practices also work on a neurological level. The awareness gained through these practices in regards to your thoughts and feelings also plays a vital role in how your body functions. Imagine going straight back into your skull from the spot between your eyebrows and you'll come across an organ called the hypothalamus. *The hypothalamus is often referred to as the site of Mind-Body connection because it takes in data, interprets it, and then directs actions in the body based on what it perceives.*

The hypothalamus constantly monitors what is happening in the body. Taking in data related to hormone levels in the blood and neural circuitry, it identifies and balances the physical environment by stimulating the release and development of hormones[2]. Its most closely related structure in doing this is the pituitary gland.

As the hypothalamus picks up data, say the need for more thyroid hormone, it sends a hormone to the pituitary gland which instructs it to wake up the thyroid and make more thyroid hormone. When the hypothalamus gets information saying that the thyroid has indeed balanced itself back out, the hypothalamus tells everyone to chill out and stop production.

With our thoughts, we get a very similar scenario. Under fear, anger, or stress we send information to the hypothalamus that will then create a physical reality (in the sense of hormones) based on that condition. Those hormones then literally build the body based on that bit of data....fear, anger, or stress[3]. Your thoughts have now become "things" in physical form.

Why is this important? Do you want a body built of fear, anger, or stress? Or would you rather build a physical form out of love, peace, and joy? Where do you think freedom, vitality, and vibrancy come from? How about disease and inflammation?

Often we go through life completely unaware of the subtle thoughts and feelings that are constantly passing through us. We are taught to fight off sadness, hide our anger in silence or burst out in rage, shield ourselves from negativity, and ignore feelings of jealousy. We work so hard at shutting out the feelings we don't want, that we actually give them power and in doing so create a body built from negative hormonal messages.

Meditation and prayer are unique ways of identifying and understanding these thoughts and emotions. They provide time of contemplation and deep recognition of the real story that's running our lives. It takes some courage and understanding to handle and interpret some of this information, but considering the impact that it has on both your mental and physical wellbeing it probably deserves the attention.

We understand that there may be some connotations around meditation and prayer that may have you prefer one method over another. From our point of view, they are one and the same simply given different names. But that shouldn't bear any significance on how you view a practice of self-awareness and connectedness with God and fellow man.

Here is a very basic exercise to work with this practice. Sit in a comfortable chair as straight as you can. Gently close your eyes and take a deep breath using the belly breath we've discussed. See if you can focus on your breathing only. Clear your mind and focus on nothing but the inhale and exhale of your breath.

Try this for one minute right now......

First question, did you actually stop? And if you did….. what did you notice? For every single person we've ever personally spoken with about this practice they have all noticed that the mind has a tendency to run wild. Thoughts of what to do for dinner, is the laundry done, what's that funny smell, my nose itches, and more come flooding up. This is just a sample of what's going on in your head ALL the time. You have gained awareness of what you're thoughts are doing even when you're *not consciously thinking them!*

Armed with this information, you can understand why your body behaves the way it does. If you are aware of the feelings and thoughts of stress constantly bombarding your brain then you know one reason why shedding those last ten pounds is so hard. You'll understand why you're neck muscles are always so sore and why you can never sleep. You have become conscious of the "inner game" that was wreaking havoc on your waistline.

Now, you can change your game plan and win. With grace, forgiveness, and a heap of love you can alter those patterns to create new ones that heal the body. And you do it by simply choosing to. But as you can imagine, there is some depth to this practice and it often takes time to feel comfortable. Having said that, we can assure you that even fleeting moments of peace have profound impact.

We teach meditations on how to shift focus towards healing the body. And while these few lines are not adept at the full depth of the practice, here's a sample of how it works.

Choose a memory that brings up ultimate peace, joy, or love. It could be a child's hug, grandchildren playing, the touch of a significant other, an aspect of nature like a fresh snowfall, or anything that personally makes you feel ultimately at ease. *Notice in your body where you feel it.* Does it make your hands tingle? Does your heart flutter? Do you get a warm sensation through your chest? Do you see light or get excited?

That feeling you get in those moments is healing in that it sends information to your hypothalamus saying "I feel love." Your hypothalamus takes that input and creates a hormonal response to love that nourishes and heals the body. By consciously taking moments to actively choose these healing emotional states, you flip the body's physiology to one of healing and wholeness[4]. You win the inner game of healing that sheds pounds, boosts energy, and clears thinking.

It is a simple practice with profound results. You have to try it, and feel it, to know it will work. But we can assure you from personal experience and the stories shared from others, the effect of meditation and prayer are nothing short of astounding.

Meditate, pray, relax

Simple Health Action Steps

1. Take 5 minutes today to sit quietly and focus inward on your breath or on your body.

2. Notice the string of thoughts that come rushing through your mind and recognize how they may be doing this throughout your day manifesting as your physical form.

3. Follow the practice of choosing memories that are loving, thankful, peaceful, and joyful. Start establishing that practice as a regular routine to soothe your stress and create a strong, vibrant body built on positive thoughts and emotions.

Chapter 19

Our Secret Weapon.....Spices

If there is one ridiculously simple change you can make to fight cancer, lose weight, control diabetes, and improve heart function, it would be using spices. The myriad of sweet, spicy, and savory supplements we add to our food to enhance the flavor are also profoundly helpful in regards to our health.

Having had the opportunity to teach culinary students learning to become trained chefs, we were amazed at how much they learned to rely on salt as their major spice. And that makes sense considering we learned that salt is used as our primary flavor enhancer, bringing out other flavors in a dish. But we were rather surprised to discover that they didn't learn how important it is to lather on the variety of other spices.

Cooking at home you have this opportunity. You can put in as much oregano, basil, pepper, cinnamon, nutmeg, garlic or ginger as you could possibly want. You can match it to fit exactly what tastes best to you. Not only does your food taste better, but the health benefits are amazing. Here are a few examples.

> *Spices have been one of our secret weapons for lasting health. Loaded with a plethora of blood purifying, cancer fighting phytonutrients, they add taste and nutrition.*

Did you know that black pepper can help with weight loss[1]? Crushing whole peppercorn in your peppermill releases a compound found in the shell that is a major aid in weight loss. It stimulates the metabolism and aids in breaking down and melting away fat cells. Pepper is widely used in nearly every meal in our house not only because of its health benefits, but because it provides a pop and flare to our food. Instead of adding more salt to our meals we tend to add more pepper. The result is a slightly spicy effect with robust flavor that doesn't carry a massive salt load into our bodies and instead activates fat burning processes.

Were you aware that cinnamon helps control blood sugar[2]? Cinnamon contains the mineral chromium which is a powerful regulator for your blood sugar levels. This is critical for folks who suffer from diabetes. There is not a single sweet food we make in the house, from muffins to cookies to oatmeal, that doesn't have cinnamon. Like pepper, cinnamon adds another layer of flavor to the food. By adding cinnamon, we've found we are able to reduce the amount of sugar we need to use. It seems to enhance the sweetness of whatever sugar is there and allows us to use much less than is often asked for in recipes.

Did you know that powerful antioxidants capable of reducing inflammation and potentially even killing cancer cells are found in the little green flakes of basil, oregano, cilantro, mint, and parsley[2]? These herbs, used in a huge variety of foods, have a number of health benefits. Many contain cancer fighting antioxidants while others have the ability to chelate (bind and remove) toxic metals floating around the body. They can be used in any number of foods including spaghetti sauce, salsa, stir-fry, fish and chicken, and pizza. One of our favorites is to add oregano and basil to scrambled or fried eggs served with mushrooms and spinach. It packs a punch of savory flavor that really pleases the taste buds.

Had you heard about the powerful anti-inflammatory properties found within turmeric and ginger[2]? These two powdery types of spices are both known to contain compounds with the ability to drastically lower inflammation in the body. While turmeric contains the nutrient curcumin that strongly reduces inflammatory chemicals in the body, ginger has been used for centuries as a natural soothing herb for stomach upset and nausea[3,4]. Growing up in Michigan I remember being given small sips of a soda called Vernor's when I had an upset stomach. The soda contained trace amounts of ginger that helped calm the nausea and discomfort. We use ginger and turmeric primarily in stir-fry at our house. But turmeric doesn't have a strong flavor and we sneak it into other foods. Ginger gets added in smaller amounts to some other treats including oatmeal. Our best recommendation for both of these spices is to experiment with them and see how you can use them to your taste and health benefit.

Spices are a very simple way to boost both flavor and your health. *They are easy to work with, relatively inexpensive, and give you great benefit for the small amount you need to use.* Adding a variety of spices into the many different meals we prepare at home has been one of the most beneficial things we've done. Our food is so good we often find eating out dull and tasteless. At the same time we avoid a lot of low quality food while supplying our bodies with nutrients that have a wide range of benefits.

For whatever reason, people seem to not take advantage of spices. That's why we call it our Secret Weapon. It's so easy and so beneficial that most people quickly overlook it. Don't make that mistake. Play with these spices, try different combinations, and figure out how they can be part of every meal. It may just be what you were needing to boost your weight loss, fight off inflammation, control your sugar levels, or even battle cancer.

Our secret weapon, spices

Simple Health Action Steps

1. Add black pepper into your dinner tonight instead of adding more salt. If eating out, avoid dumping on more salt and try the pepper instead.

2. Put cinnamon in your next round of cookies or muffins. See if you can lower the sugar needed by about a $1/8^{th}$ of a cup.

3. Experiment with the variety of spices and herbs available to you. See what works well together and suits your tastes. You can look up information on their particular health benefits and then create your own combos to suit your health goals as well.

Chapter 20

Get Moving! But for goodness sakes....HAVE FUN!

We all know we should exercise. But why do so many of us not do it? Very often we don't exercise because it seems like some miserable responsibility. We loathe having to spend time on a treadmill or hate going into a gym with intimidating trainers and meat-heads. But exercise can be as simple as anything else. You just need to start moving.

My mother was adamant about not exercising. She said she hated to sweat. Despite having children who were involved in all sorts of exercise and sports, she didn't want anything to do with it. It turned out her primary concern was that she wasn't comfortable with exercise because she'd never known *how* to exercise. What moves work certain muscles? How much weight do you use? How far should I walk and how fast should I be going? What can I do if I don't like doing that exercise or following this certain plan? These are all common questions that rarely get voiced and keep people afraid of getting started.

Fortunately for my mom, she joined a corporate challenge on a whim and found herself trying things she'd never considered. With a little instruction she found herself enjoying yoga, going on evening walks, and eventually joining the gym! It's hard to express how big of a step this was.

Just three years later she was used as a spotlight success story for her local gym as a shining example of what changes can be made, and how amazing you can feel, if you just start doing something.

What was the key? She had to enjoy it. It had to be something that provided a reward and wasn't boring or painful. The last thing she wanted to do was sit around a bunch of machines counting reps and watching an hour pass by. She needed to be engaged and active. Doing one set and waiting for two minutes was repetitive and dull and quickly lost her interest.

How many people go to the gym and pound out a few miles on the treadmill mindlessly plugging along so bored they have to cover up the display so they can't see how long they have left? We can relate and would bet you've known this problem, too.

It's important to enjoy what you're doing anywhere, especially at the gym. Any time exercise gets stagnant and dull for us we switch it up. As mentioned before we use yoga and Muay Thai as great changes of pace. Maybe you take a dance class with your significant other. Make family bike rides a regular evening event. Play on a co-ed soccer or softball team. Walk in the park or join a group in the mall. Experiment with finding exercises on YouTube. Maybe you'll find something you really like and that gets you excited about moving and being active. When exercise becomes less of a chore and turns into something you look forward to, the opportunity for quick, healthy changes accelerates exponentially. You get better results faster.

> *Hours on a treadmill bored to tears is pointless. For real fat-melting, muscle-toning results make your workouts fun!*

Once my mom found her groove, the weight started coming off easily. She found herself excited about workouts and felt amazing with all her added energy. She noticed that she was able to do more and be more engaged in her home life. My mom even rode down a zip line and climbed a rock wall with us at a family reunion! Nothing seemed impossible and life was really being lived. We recognized my mom had been living in a shell. Watching her break free has been one of the most exciting times of my life. And I know it has been transformational for her.

Yes, exercise is important. Just like eating, breathing, relaxing, loving, forgiving, and everything else. But it doesn't have to be misery. In fact, it should be fun! The experiences and freedom that come with it are life-altering.

Just recently I started training a gentleman whose workouts have been dull, erratic, and ineffective. He's committed to feeling the energy and vitality that he knows is possible for his mind and body. He is aware that the days of football are over. But he also knows that the feeling of aliveness is not. We didn't do anything crazy or overly exciting. We just started by taking ordinary exercises he usually did separately and strung them together in a creative, engaging way. Even though the pace and intensity were challenging, I could see that the confidence and willingness to continue started with that first step.

One of the important statements he made was that the workouts at the pace and level we did them were fun. He had resisted gym memberships and exercise plans because boredom always seemed to derail his efforts. It's a story we hear all the time. But it doesn't have to be the case.

Start with a single step. It's not necessary to run off and join the gym right away. Moving and starting this journey can be done working in the garden 30 minutes every day or taking the dog for a 30 minute walk every day. Rent a video from the library on yoga, Pilates, or Zumba. Take the drying laundry off the exercise machine in your house and give it a whirl while you watch TV. It doesn't matter where you start, it just matters that you do and that you have fun doing it.

Get moving

Simple Health Action Steps

1. Make moving a regular part of your day by making it something you enjoy. If you don't want to spend an hour in the gym, don't. Work in your garden, play with your kids or grandkids, or rent a video and exercise at home.

2. Keep changing things up. Stave off boredom and keep moving forward by trying new exercises and challenging yourself in different ways.

3. Once you're comfortable, join a group exercise class or sports team. Working out with and around people becomes a lot of fun and pushes you a little extra helping propel you further towards your goals.

Chapter 21

Take Baby Steps

Growing up in Northern Michigan my family would take our yearly summer vacation to visit my relatives in Chicago. During the drive we always used the same landmarks. There was the big bend and pointed church steeple in Grand Rapids, the merge onto an actual expressway in the city of Cadillac, the "Chicago – 99 Miles" sign and of course our first view of the skyline telling us we were close.

My parents were smart in breaking the long trip down into smaller baby steps. With each landmark we felt the reward of progress and were excited to reach the next one. When looking at what it takes to reach transformations in health, following the same pattern is wise advice.

This may not be what you want to hear. The idea of making sweeping changes that radically alter everything about your health and your life is far more enticing. But in reality, they are rarely practical and often don't lead to long-term success.

While losing seven pounds in seven days sounds awesome, it might not be right for you. What is hidden in those messages is that often these fantastic weight loss ideas are built around temporary success with long term misery. Win today, lose tomorrow. The mere cycle of dieting for rapid, massive weight loss destroys your metabolism, interrupts your body's physiology, and creates a major problem for how your body will react to healthy efforts later[1,2]. Most dieters do not have true fat loss. Instead they shed water weight and destroy lean muscle tissue, setting them up for immediate weight gain once they go off the diet.

Likewise, going overboard at the gym leads to injury. Or cutting out all the guilty pleasures at once makes life agony and you quickly "fall off the wagon."

That's why real success, sustained over time, comes with taking baby steps. Yes, sometimes drastic overhauls are needed. There's been times we've had to completely clear out pantries of coaching clients and basically start all over. But even then, rarely is it a complete transformation in one swoop. It takes time and some energy at first. You have to walk before you can run. And trying to do too much, too fast can set you back.

Having big goals divided into smaller increments provides time for rewards. You get a positive neurochemical flush of dopamine, the happy hormone, when you reach your first weight loss goal or go a day without a candy bar. The reactions that happen in the brain create neural circuitry that actively seeks out further rewards gained by doing healthy actions. As you repeat the process and attain more rewards by achieving more goals, the brain continually builds patterns of further reward. In the end, you build an entire brain that is attuned to creating positive changes.

Weight loss is a wonderful example of this concept. Since so many people have a desire to shed weight, there's no shortage of "experts" promoting their sure-fire therapies for drastic results in unbelievable time without having to do any work. But as mentioned before, this is neither healthy nor effective.

Setting positive goals for weight loss that have been shown to have consistent, long term impact involves breaking it down into smaller goals that move towards an overall big dream. Let's say you're eighty pounds overweight. You set an intention that you will lose those eighty pounds and when New Year's Day hits you get started. How will you track your progress? How will you know if you're on pace to lose the full eighty in that year or are only on track to lose fifty?

You do this by setting smaller goals that act as landmarks. If you want to lose 80 pounds you could set up goals to lose seven pounds a month. (80 pounds divided by 12 months roughly equates to seven pounds a month) That doesn't sound like much but it also sounds and feels more doable and achievable. Your mind can grasp losing seven pounds far more easily than it can eighty. You'll also be able to measure if you're on target to reach your goal at the end of each month or determine if you've gotten stuck in a rut and need to make changes. You can track success over the course of many months to plan ahead and create a detailed map of where you're heading. If March was tough and you lost only five pounds maybe you can just lose one extra pound in April and May.

Using this strategy simultaneously removes some of the stress and urgency often felt around big goals, both of which sabotage weight loss. (Remember stress triggers fight or flight systems in the body that over time store fat and wear down the body.) You'll have to consider consistent long term choices that provide continual benefit. You'll have to avoid quick fixes and fads or learn on the fly what works and what doesn't. Soon enough, you'll discover for yourself that steady, positive growth using tools like addition before subtraction are far more effective than cleverly named gimmicks.

There is one potential setback to be aware of here. It is possible to set too small of goals in too short increments of time. For example, you don't want to step on the scale and check your weight every day, or even every week. The emotional toll that comes with minimal ups and downs is really scary. Seeing a number on the scale go up or not change for three straight days is often more damaging than the positive impact of seeing that number going down. Laying the plan out over a month and waiting for that time to measure your progress (at least every two weeks) is far more enabling when it comes to reaching the ultimate goal. You have to walk before you can run, but we don't want to regress back to crawling either.

Most goals are best set out with a yearly intention broken down into monthly baby steps. Certainly, we encourage you to have 5-year, 10-year, even 20 or 50-year plans. Each of those should be accompanied by *specific action steps you can do right now with smaller goals along the way to know your progress.* Put these in places you will see them consistently and do something each day that acts towards those goals. Keep yourself action-oriented so that you make progress and avoid being stuck on the hamster wheel. If you get off course, just get right back on. Forgive yourself, love yourself, and begin again.

Take baby steps

Simple Health Action Steps

1. Break down your overall big goal into monthly smaller goals. If you want to run a marathon, set a plan for how you will build up to running 26.2 miles. You'll probably start by running 3!

2. Track your progress monthly (maybe every 2 weeks) to avoid the plague of feeling like you're going nowhere by not seeing change every single day.

3. If you get off course, regroup, refresh and begin again. It may mean you need to re-evaluate and change some things you're doing. But make the change and get right back to it.

BONUS

The Amazingly Awesome, Super Cool Power of Compassion

At a recent meeting we heard a woman give a short speech about her struggles with weight loss. Around a year earlier she had given birth to her first child and was struggling with letting go of the "baby weight." She had been trying diets, putting in new workouts, and reading books with advice that sometimes got really strange. None of it worked.

Then she shared the missing piece she had discovered. Compassion and confidence for herself. A willingness to be okay with who she is and what she wants for herself. And the self-love to recognize that this goal of weight loss was more for honoring herself than it was for fitting into a societal box.

Suddenly, in nine months she lost nearly 55 pounds. She said the weight and frustration both just seemed to start flushing away with far more ease than she had ever imagined. With the weight going she noticed that she had more energy for family, school, and work. She was happier and felt she could be more authentic with those around her. And it gave her the confidence to stand up in front of a room of people she hardly knew and share a story that involved personal vulnerability around a deep hurt that ended with a glorious triumph.

> *There's a mental and emotional aspect of weight loss and healing that is just as important as all the physical tools you utilize.*

Compassion for ourselves and others is one of the most challenging concepts to grasp. Even if we are often excellent at showing compassion towards friends, relatives, or perfect strangers, we somehow bind ourselves with the inability to easily and freely show compassion for ourselves. The judgments we make about our looks, careers, intelligence, accomplishments, finances, and many more act like mental weights we carry around like boulders on our backs. We hide them, even from ourselves, and pretend like they're not there. But we also are keenly aware of their burden whenever they arise.

Shifting into a state of compassion for ourselves is sometimes harder than any physical change we can make. Why? Because while we can measure how much water we drink or how many servings of vegetables we had yesterday, measuring our level of compassion and self-care is nearly impossible to do. How can you determine if you love yourself more today than yesterday? And what does it mean when you have one good day followed by two bad ones and then four more great days of loving compassion? What does progress look like?

Here are signs for you to use as a means of performing a "check-in" to know if you're living and acting with more compassion for yourself and others.

First, you experience more patience and forgiveness. Showing compassion often means recognizing that we're all doing the best we can at the level we're at. There's no secret formula for life that everyone must follow and we should have individual goals, dreams, and means of getting there. Think of rush hour traffic. Everyone is trying to get to their respective destinations in the fastest way possible. But sometimes there are people who view their particular journeys as more important. So they weave in and out of cars, rush into merging lanes, causing a cascade of brake lights effectively slowing traffic further.

Compassion during rush hour can look like you allowing someone who needs to get in your lane a spot to move over. It can mean making the necessary moves yourself to be in position for your exit early instead of having to fight through three or four lanes within a quarter mile. You show patience for everyone who is doing exactly what you're doing.

Rush hour traffic is much like life. We are all trying to get where we want to be....experiencing happiness, freedom, peace, and love. And while the destinations may look different for each of us, we are all doing our best to get there amidst the sea of others doing the same. Compassion for each person, and for yourself, recognizes the similarities of the road you're traveling, and respects the differences. Understanding your journey is just like someone else's (though it may look different) creates patience and allows you to forgive as you would hope to be forgiven. And yes, with deeper compassion you have greater patience for yourself and deeper forgiveness for yourself as well.

Second, *compassion shows up as honoring yourself.* How do you know if you're honoring yourself? Because the things that you're doing make you feel good and inspire confidence. You have a level of self-satisfaction that you ate a big salad at lunch, skipped the donuts, and went for a walk when you got home from work. You let the criticism of a co-worker or the angry honk from a fellow driver roll off your back and even showed patience towards them in the process.

Honoring yourself mentally, emotionally, and physically is easy to know because it shows up as energy and lightness in the body. Positive steps in your nutrition, exercise, thoughts, feelings, water consumption, etc. are all easily identified because there's more energy, more joy, more love, and more optimism.

When you're feeling doubtful, irritated, and pessimistic about your choices; you are simply getting information telling you that you've chosen options that are not for your highest good. They are merely measuring sticks to inform you of where you are in relation to where you want to be. Deeper compassion means recognizing this distinction and moving back into that which honors you further.

Third, you relax, live in the moment, and be authentically you. One of the greatest tools of self-sabotage is replaying our failures in our minds or projecting them onto the future. *Compassion allows you to move beyond the regrets of yesterday and the fears of tomorrow by putting you squarely in the moment.*

You're relaxed, aware, at ease, and looking forward to life. You enjoy what shows up for you even if it shows up as pizza or drinks with friends when your "diet" won't allow it. But the key is that doing so with compassion means you won't kick yourself later for the fun and joy you had in those moments. It recognizes that pizza with joy is better than a salad with remorse and pity.

However, it also means being able to say "no" in the moment as well. There is tremendous power in "No." In that relaxed state of personal knowing, you consciously choose what is best for you. That may mean eating pizza, or not. It may mean hanging out with friends and never ordering a drink. You are relaxed and in the moment as yourself with the self-compassion that allows you to make the best choice for you....whatever it may be.

The more you are relaxed, in the moment, and authentically being yourself, the more you are expressing compassion.

We know this concept seems somewhat out there and "new-age." It's hard to discuss or even get into any depth in just a few paragraphs. But the importance of compassion shows up every single day in our lives. However you begin to understand what compassion means or feels like, give yourself the freedom to explore and work with it.

Like the woman who had to find her confidence and compassion before she could drop those extra pounds, we know from our own experiences that deep compassion, for both ourselves and others, is key to not just reaching our goals but in finding appreciation and joy that makes life worth living.

Power of compassion

Simple Health Action Steps

1. Today work on showing compassion towards another person when they upset you. It could be someone driving, a co-worker, or even your family. Show patience and calm amidst the upset. Let the upset pass through you like a passing cloud and let it be done.

2. Notice whether you are expressing compassion for yourself by looking for the three signs: Patience and forgiveness, honoring yourself, and living authentically in the moment.

3. Find and Use an affirmation that you can recite which affirms your compassion for both yourself and others to establish the neural circuitry that creates peaceful wellness.

Resources

Chapter 1:

1.   7 Science-Based Health Benefits of Drinking Enough Water, By Joe Leech, Dietitian. July, 2015   http://authoritynutrition.com/7-health-benefits-of-water/

Chapter 2:

1.   http:createsimplehealth.com/videos

Chapter 3:

1.   http://hereandnow.wbur.org/2015/07/29/gmo-foods-debate

2.   www.organicconsumers.org/old_articles/gefood/countrieswithbans.php

3.   30-Second Food Label Scan.   Dr.   Kevin   Morford. http://createsimplehealth/videos

Chapter 4:

1.   Physiological Effects of Medium-Chain Triglycerides: Potential Agents in the Prevention of Obesity, Marie Pierre St-Onge and Peter Jones, Journal of Nutrition 132; 329-332, 2002

2.   Effects of dietary coconut oil on the biochemical and anthropometric profiles of women presenting abdominal obesity, Lipids, 2009 July; 44 (7) 593-601

3.   Weston A. Price, DDS and the Weston A. Price Foundation Dietary Guidelines

4.   Cholesterol, Coconuts, and diet on Polynesian atolls: a natural experiment; the Pukapuka and Tokelau island studies, IA Prior et al., American Journal of Clinical Nutrition, 1981 vol. 34, 1552-1561

5.   Anti-inflammatory, analgesic, and antipyretic activities of virgin coconut oil, Intahphuak S., et al. Pharmacological Biology, 2010, 48(2), 151-7

6. In vivo antinociceptive and anti-inflammatory activities of dried and fermented processed virgin coconut oil, Zakaria ZA, et al. Med Princ. Pract., 2011, 20(3)231-6

Chapter 7:

1. Your Brain and Physiology of Love. Modified on September 11, 2015 by Kaitlin Goodrich. https://www.brainscape.com/blog/2015/06/physiology-of-love/

Chapter 8:

1. www.lumosity.com

2. www.recipes.com

Chapter 9:

1. Excitotoxins: The Taste that Kills. Russell Blaylock, MD. Health Press Santa Fe, New Mexico 1997

2. www.NutraLegacy.com; Top 10 Dangers of Artificial Sweeteners

3. Artificial Sweeteners - More Dangerous than You've Ever Imagined. Dr. Joseph Mercola http://articles.mercola.com/sites/articles/archive/2009/10/13/a rtificial-sweeteners-more-dangerous-than-you-ever-imagined.aspx

4. www.medicine.net; Artificial Sweeteners

Chapter 11:

1. Nutrients in Food Colors. Dr. William Sears. http://www.askdrsears.com/topics/feeding-eating/family-nutrition/food-colors-nutritious

2. Color Me Healthy — Eating for a Rainbow of Benefits. By Juliann Schaeffer. *Today's Dietitian November 2008*   Vol. 10 No. 11 P. 34

Chapter 13:

1. www.drsuemorter.com Intentional Living Series

2. Spiritual Liberation: Fulfilling Your Souls Potential. Rev. Dr. Michael Beckwith. Atria Paperback, 2008

3. www.emdr.com

Chapter 15:

1. The Effectiveness and Cost-Effectiveness of Chiropractic Management of Low Back Pain. Manga, Pran Ph.D. et al. Funded by Ontario Ministry of Health, 1993

2. A comparison of health care costs for chiropractic and medical patients. Stano, M. J Manipulative Physiol Ther. 1993 Jun; 16(5):291-9.

Chapter 16:

1. Dr. Joseph Mercola. www.mercola.com. Fermented Foods: How to Culture Your Way to Optimal Health.

2. http://nutritionwonderland.com/2009/06/understanding-bodies-serotonin-connection-between-food-and-mood/

3. Audio from Scientific American: http://www.scientificamerican.com/podcast/episode/fecal-transplants-the-straight-poop-12-01-31/

Chapter 18:

1. Science of the Heart: Exploring the Role of the Heart in Human Performance:An Overview of Research Conducted by the HeartMath Institute

    a. https://www.heartmath.org/resources/downloads/science-of-the-heart/

2. Buddha's Brain: The Practical Neuroscience of Happiness, Love, and Wisdom. Rick Hanson, Ph.D., with Richard Mendius, MD. New Harbisher Publications, Inc. 2009

3. The Physiological and Psychological Effects of Compassion and Anger. Glen Rein, Mike Atkinson, and Rollin McCraty. Journal of Advancement in Medicine. 1995; 8(2): 87-105.

4. Cardiac Coherence, Self-Regulation, Autonomic Stability, and Psychosocial Well-Being. Rollin McCraty Ph.D.1 and Maria A Zayas2; 1 Institute of HeartMath, Boulder Creek, CA, USA. 2 Department of Psychology, Brenau University, Gainesville, GA, USA. Frontiers in Psychology, Sept. 2014. Vol. 5, Article 1090

Chapter 19:

1. https://www.organicfacts.net/health-benefits/herbs-and-spices/health-benefits-of-black-pepper.html

2. http://www.livestrong.com/article/299675-10-most-antioxidant-spices/

3. Antioxidant and anti-inflammatory properties of curcumin. Menon VP[1], Sudheer AR. Adv Exp Med Biol. 2007;595:105-25.

4. Ginger: Health Benefits, Facts, Research Written by Megan Ware RDN LD Last updated: Tue 5 January 2016 http://www.medicalnewstoday.com/articles/265990.php

Chapter 21:

1. The Effects of Diet and Metabolism on the Body. Rich Amber. http://www.naturalnews.com/022347_diet_metabolism_calories.html

2. Your Hidden Food Allergies are Making You Fat: How to Lose Weight and Gain Years of Vitality. Rudy Rivera, MD and Roger Davis Deutsch. Three Rivers Press, a part of Random House, Inc. New York, 2002

OTHER RECOMMENDED HEALTH RESOURCES:

Dr. Joseph Mercola - www.mercola.com

www.heartmath.org

Dr. Sue Morter – The Energy Codes Seminar Series

Dr. Sue Morter – Body Awake DVDs - DrSueMorter.com

Environmental Working Group - www.EWG.org

David Wolfe – www.DavidWolfe.com

Natural Awakenings Magazine

Encyclopedia of Nutritional Supplements: The Essential Guide for Improving Your Health Naturally by Michael T. Murray (Jul 24, 1996)

Food, Inc. The Movie

The Secret, Movie

Dr. Deepak Chopra – www.deepakchopra.com

About the Authors

Dr. April Morford has used simple health techniques to overcome severe childhood asthma. Through her work in nutrition and exercise she transformed from an inhaler bound sufferer to finishing the Houston Marathon. She serves as the lead science faculty at Platt College in Oklahoma City and is a member of the global organization, Wisdompreneurs. She is a Chiropractic Physician certified in the energy medicine modality BioEnergetic Synchronization Technique (B.E.S.T.).

As a doctor, teacher, wife, and mother, Dr. April balances her professional and personal life expertly. Her professional time is spent in private practice and individual coaching focusing on creating awareness and using the body's natural ability to heal itself. She has worked with clients helping them find success in a variety of health challenges ranging from weight loss to autoimmune disorders. Her work is designed to create a vibrant life by bridging health and human consciousness.

Dr. Kevin Morford has over 15 years of experience in the health and wellness industry. After starting by working in a hospital while an undergraduate student, he has continued to serve in schools, clinics, and currently maintains his private practice. He serves as an instructor at Oklahoma State University in Oklahoma City and is also a member of the global organization, Wisdompreneurs. He is a Chiropractic Physician with a certificate in Chiropractic Neurology and practices in Edmond, Oklahoma.

He spends most of his professional time between speaking and private practice. He has been a keynote speaker at various conferences and corporations. His presentations, articles, and workshops provide insight and practices into linking the body, brain, and consciousness to create daily habits that provide consistent positive change for lasting health and vitality.

Dr. April and Dr. Kevin enjoy an active lifestyle with their daughter based in Edmond, OK.

Connect with Dr. April and Dr. Kevin

For more information, services, and products from Dr. Kevin Morford and Dr. April Morford including corporate workshops and personal or small group coaching visit them at the websites below.

Dr. Kevin Morford

www.DrKevinMorford.com

facebook.com/DrKevinMorford

twitter.com/DrKevinMorford

Dr. April Morford

www.DrAprilMorford.com

facebook.com/DrAprilMorford

twitter.com/DrAprilM